ORTHOPEDIC NURSING

ORTHOPEDIC NURSING

CLARA A. DONAHOO, R.N.
Orthopedic Nurse Specialist

JOSEPH H. DIMON III, M.D.
Orthopedic Surgeon
Both at the Peachtree Orthopedic Clinic
Atlanta, Georgia

LITTLE, BROWN AND COMPANY
Boston

Library of Congress Catalog Card No. 76-52626

ISBN 0-316-18940-5

Printed in the United States of America

PREFACE

It has been our intent to present clearly and concisely material that is pertinent in the daily practice of orthopedic nursing. Although the text is designed primarily for the orthopedic nurse-practitioner, it will be of value to nursing students as well as those nurses re-entering the profession in this specialty.

This text on orthopedic nursing is intended to be a supplementary text or reference book dealing only with the nursing care of those patients with known or suspected diseases or conditions of the neuromusculoskeletal system. Because the specialty of orthopedics encompasses so many recognized modes of treatment, we have limited our discussion to the clinical problems most frequently encountered. The psychosocial aspects of orthopedic nursing have not been dealt with in detail, and we would refer the reader to specialized books on this subject for more information.

We realize that a nurse caring for an orthopedic patient must first have a basic understanding of the principles of nursing practice as well as clinical expertise in caring for patients. This book was written for nurses with these fundamental skills.

The specialty of orthopedics is constantly changing, as is the nursing care of patients. We have presented the current concepts of treatment and nursing care. Although techniques and equipment may vary geographically, the underlying principles are the same.

We would like to think of this book as a testimonial to our basic conviction that orthopedic surgeons and orthopedic nurses can and should work closely together to improve the quality of care of the orthopedic patient.

We acknowledge the outstanding assistance of King Dasher in the preparation of photographic materials used in this text. The drawings were expertly rendered by George DeGrazio of Idaho Springs, Colorado.

C. A. D.
J. H. D.
Atlanta

CONTENTS

ORTHOPEDIC
NURSING

1. NURSING ASSESSMENT

N ursing assessment is the collection of information concerning the patient through interview, physical examination, and review of records and reports.

HISTORY
All nursing histories should include the patient's medical diagnosis and therapy, past history, allergies, social habits, family history, and review of symptoms. There are certain areas of the interview history which, although pertinent with any patient, need elaboration for the person with a known or suspected neuromusculoskeletal alteration. Special attention is given to the history taken at the interview, as described in this section, since this information will be helpful in identifying neuromusculoskeletal injuries or disease processes by the causative factors, associated loss of function, or pain patterns.

It is important to know the *onset of symptoms* or the *mechanism* and *time of injury*. A careful history of the *progression of the symptoms* and *limitation of function* due to these symptoms should be recorded.

The orthopedic patient may have a variety of symptoms, but the nurse must be careful to obtain an accurate description of pain, weakness, numbness, or loss of function. These complaints are most important in the overall evaluation of a patient with a known or suspected orthopedic disease or condition. One must consider the entire symptom complex and the entire course rather than just the primary complaint.

To say that the patient has pain is inadequate; one must describe the quality or character of the pain and numbness or radiation associated with the pain. It is also important to document any limitation of motion that may be associated with the pain. Other factors to be considered are the time of occurrence or known causative factors. Many patients are able to obtain relief from pain by use of external supports, position, or medications; this information must be obtained and recorded.

Although the pharmacologic history is obtained for all patients, the interviewer must obtain information from all orthopedic patients, especially concerning their *previous use of steroids*. Most physicians now feel that any patient who has previously received steroids, regardless of the time element, should receive steroid coverage for any surgery.

PHYSICAL ASSESSMENT

The physical examination is a part of the nursing assessment, although many nurses feel that this is not within the scope of nursing practice. The physical examination is more systematic when divided into *general assessment* and *orthopedic assessment* of the patient.

The normal versus the abnormal *general appearance* of an individual is discussed in many texts. The subject will not be belabored here, except to say that concurrently and recurrently the nurse caring for an orthopedic patient must be particularly aware of pressure points, skin petechiae, calf tenderness, and localized edema, since these findings are often pertinent to the patient's care.

The *orthopedic physical assessment* is essential not only in determining the diagnosis, but also in documenting the patient's progress and evaluating any permanent disability. The tools required are one's eyes, ears, hands, and a basic knowledge of norms. The accessory tools are a tape measure, a reflex hammer, a goniometer, and a safety pin. The nurse frequently sees the patient in a different setting and in a greater variety of situations than does the physician. These opportunities should be utilized to observe the patient when he or she is unaware. During this time the nurse may observe the overall position and appearance of the trunk and extremities. Apparent normal growth and development should also be noted.

Mobility in getting into or out of bed or a chair should be noted, as well as gait in an ambulatory patient. Use of external supports should be documented.

A basic understanding of *normal gait* is helpful to the nurse in evaluating gait abnormalities. When a person is standing, the weight of the body is evenly distributed on the two lower extremities; this is considered the normal stance. When walking forward, the left leg is advanced so that it is no longer touching the floor and all the body weight is transmitted to the right leg. The right leg is going through what is called a stance phase, supporting the body weight. As the left leg is brought forward and placed down on the floor, the first thing that happens is that the left heel strikes the floor; this is called the heel strike. The foot is then plantar flexed and the weight is gradually shifted from the stance phase, the weight bearing phase, of the right foot to the left lower extremity. Push-off occurs when the individual pushes off with the foot from the stance phase, the weight is borne on the forefoot, the heel comes off the ground, and the body is propelled forward. Push-off requires strong plantar flexion of the foot. The transmission of weight bearing from one extremity to another occurs in a predictable, smooth, and easy fashion unless there is abnormality in the joints or muscles. When an individual stands on just one leg the center of gravity of the body falls medial to the hip joint of the stance leg. This position tends to make the pelvis drop down on the non-stance side. This force is balanced and the pelvis is held level by a contraction of the abductor muscles that run from the iliac portion of the pelvis to the greater trochanter of the stance hip. These muscles have to be contracted forcefully to hold the pelvis stable (approximate force of 2.5 times body weight). If for any reason there is pain in the hip joint or the abductor muscles do not function normally, a smooth balancing mechanism is absent and an abnormal gait will be noticed; the patient will swing the shoulders over the affected hip joint so that the center of gravity of the body drops through the hip joint, relieving the necessity of contracting the abductor muscles. These patients have what is called a shoulder-shift weight bearing gait, or abductor lurch.

If the quadriceps muscle cannot be normally contracted (because of paralysis, pain in the knee with use, and so forth) during the stance phase of gait, the knee will bend and the patient will fall unless he or she (1) keeps the center of gravity in front of the knee joint, thereby tightening the posterior knee joint capsule, which locks the knee in hypertension, or (2) plants the extremity in a plane that allows the joint to be stable without contracting the quadriceps. The patient accomplishes (1) by leaning forward over the knee when bearing weight on the affected side, or by pushing the thigh with a hand in order to keep the center of gravity in front of the knee. He or she accomplishes (2) by externally rotating the knee so that the bending force occurs in line with the medial collateral ligament, which is strong and will not allow the knee to give way in that particular plane.

If the presenting problem involves a joint, the *joint motion* must be measured and recorded. In order to record the findings in a language that will be understood by others, one must become familiar with the terms of joint range of motion. The terms used in the measurement and definition of joint range of motion include the following:

Adduction — movement of the limb toward the body center
Abduction — movement away from midline of the body
Extension — straightening out of the joint (extremity)
Hyperextension — extension beyond the ordinary range
Pronation — turning downward (palm), turning downward and outward (foot)
Supination — turning upward (palm), turning upward and inward (foot)

Flexion — bending of a joint (extremity)

Dorsiflexion — lifting foot up toward shin (ankle), lifting fingers and wrist up (hand)

Plantar flexion — pushing foot down (ankle), bending fingers and wrist down toward palm (hand)

Rotation — turning or movement of a part around its axis

Internal — turning inward toward the center

External — turning outward away from the center

Eversion — turning the foot outward

Inversion — turning the foot toward the midline

Radial deviation — movement of the hand toward the radius

Ulnar deviation — movement of the hand toward the ulna

Varus — abnormal deviation toward the midline of the alignment of the extremity distal to the joint or point of reference in the coronal plane

Valgus — abnormal deviation away from the midline of the alignment of the extremity distal to the joint or point of reference in the coronal plane

The neutral (anatomic) position of any joint is 0 degrees. Flexion, extension, adduction, abduction, internal rotation, external rotation, supination and pronation (pertain to forearm only), and radial and ulnar deviation (pertain to wrist only) are all measured from this starting point of 0 degrees. If the elbow or knee normally extends past this neutral position, its placement should be termed hyperextension; similarly, the inability to assume the neutral position should be recorded as a flexion deformity.

All joint motions must be identified as right or left and recorded in degrees; it should be noted whether active or passive motion has been measured. A goniometer is an instrument used to measure joint position and motion (Fig. 1-1). It is used at the elbow, for example, by placing the center of the instrument over the axis of the joint with its arms in line with the bones on each side of the joint, the elbow being in maximum extension. The position of the joint is read on the goniometer. The elbow is then maximally flexed and the new joint position is read and recorded.

The neutral position of the shoulder is with the arm at the side, the elbow extended, and the forearm in the neutral position. The shoulder is a complex joint and can move in many planes (Fig. 1-2). Even if the glenohumeral joint is stiff, motion between the scapula and chest can give overall motion of the arm and the ability to lift the arm out to the side. The position of internal rotation is with the forearm across the body, and external rotation is movement of the forearm on the shoulder axis out to the side. The ability to raise the arm overhead, straight out to the side, is combined abduction, and

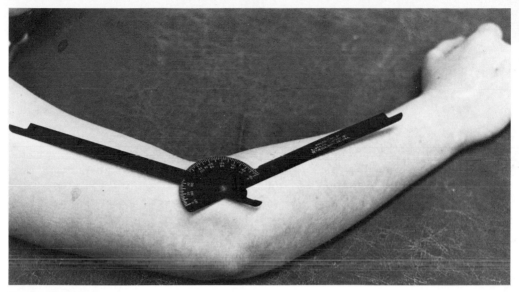

Figure 1-1. A go-
niometer is used
to measure elbow
joint motion.

Figure 1-2. Range
of motion in the
shoulder.

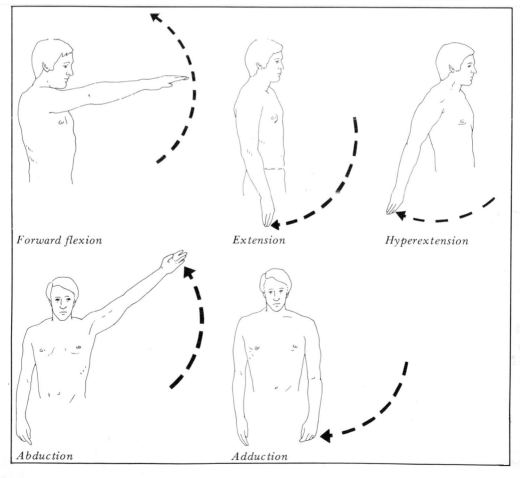

Forward flexion

Extension

Hyperextension

Abduction

Adduction

the ability to do this by raising the arm forward is flexion. From a practical standpoint, the nurse should note the ability or lack of ability of the patient to put the hand behind the back; (limited internal rotation is an early sign of pericapsulitis); the ability of the patient to rotate the arm out to the side; (limited external rotation may be a sign of posterior shoulder dislocation or capsulitis); and the patient's ability or inability to raise the arm overhead (which may indicate painful joint, rotator cuff injury, bursitis, or paralysis).

The elbow is in a neutral, or 0-degree, position when it is absolutely straight. If the elbow extends past this neutral position, it is in hyperextension, also referred to as recurvatum. Flexion of the elbow is determined by measuring the number of degrees between the upper arm and the forearm with the elbow completely bent (Fig. 1-3). A flexion deformity of the elbow (elbow does not fully extend) is determined by measuring the number of degrees between the upper arm and the forearm with the elbow in maximum extension.

The forearm is in a neutral, or 0-degree, position when the arm is at the side, the elbow flexed to 90 degrees, and the forearm in a position with the back of the thumb facing up. Pronation and supination are the ability of the patient to turn the palm up (supination) or down (pronation) (Fig. 1-3). These motions can be accomplished by the shoulder; therefore, the evaluation is valid only when measurements are taken with the elbows fixed at the side.

The wrist is in a neutral position when the palm is facing down and the radius and metacarpals are in a straight plane (Fig. 1-4). Dorsiflexion is the motion of raising (extending) the entire hand up as far as possible past the neutral position, and palmar flexion is bending the hand down from the wrist past the neutral position; in both cases the number of degrees between the forearm and metacarpals is recorded. Ulnar deviation is the motion of the hand from the wrist to the outside (ulnar side) of the arm and is measured as the number of degrees between the long finger metacarpal and the forearm. Radial deviation is the motion of the hand from the wrist to the inside (radial side) of the arm and is also measured as the number of degrees between the long finger metacarpal and the forearm (Figs. 1-5, 1-6).

The hip is in a neutral, or 0-degree, position when the thigh is aligned with the trunk in all planes. Measurements are generally performed with the patient supine. Flexion of the hip is determined by bringing the thigh as close to the trunk as it will go, allowing the knee to bend (Fig. 1-7). The number of degrees between the thigh and the trunk represents hip flexion. Abduction is the movement of the hip away from the midline. It is measured from the neutral joint position and

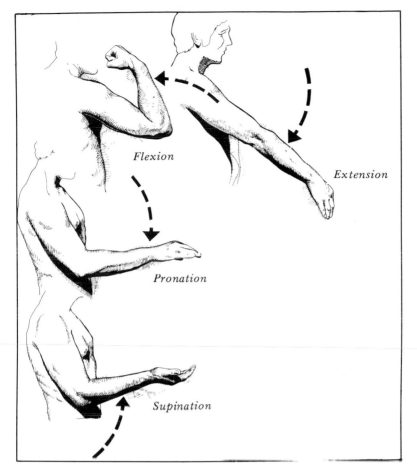

Flexion

Extension

Pronation

Supination

Figure 1-3. Range of motion in the elbow.

Figure 1-4. Range of motion in the wrist.

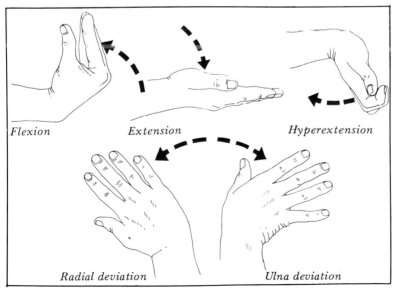

Flexion

Extension

Hyperextension

Radial deviation

Ulna deviation

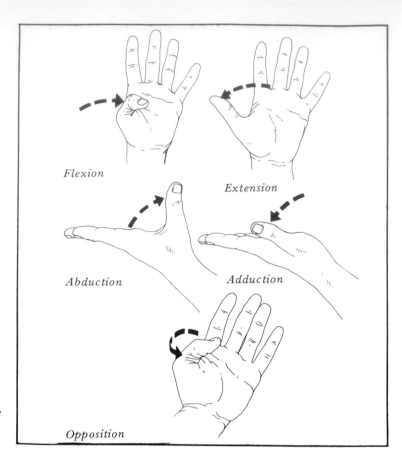

Flexion

Extension

Abduction

Adduction

Opposition

Figure 1-5. Range of motion in the thumb.

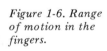

Figure 1-6. Range of motion in the fingers.

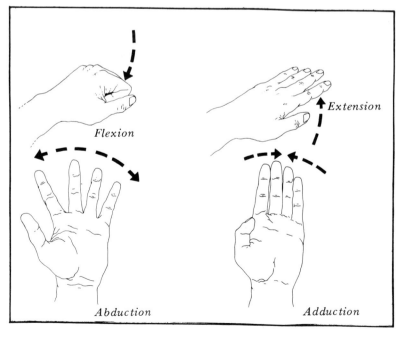

Flexion

Extension

Abduction

Adduction

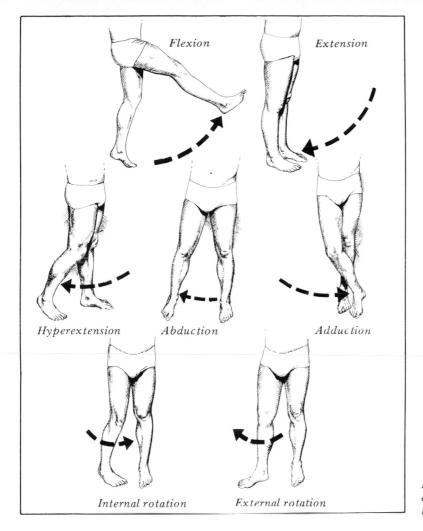

Figure 1-7. Range
of motion in the
hip.

may be recorded as abduction (number of degrees) in flexion
or abduction in extension. Adduction is the movement of the
thigh toward the midline. It is measured from the neutral
joint position and may be recorded as adduction (number of
degrees) in flexion or adduction in extension. Internal rotation is a measurement of the number of degrees that the hip
will rotate toward the midline from the neutral position. It
may be measured both in flexion and in extension. External
rotation is a measurement of the number of degrees that the
hip will rotate away from the midline from the neutral position and may also be measured both in flexion and in extension. A flexion contracture of the hip is demonstrated by first
flexing the opposite hip toward the trunk, so that the back
and pelvis are flat on the examining table. If the thigh lies on

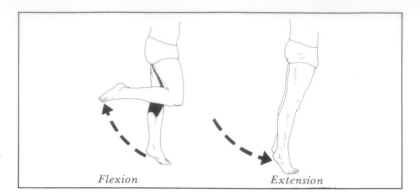

Figure 1-8. Range of motion in the knee.

Flexion   Extension

the table surface there is no flexion contracture present. If it does not extend all the way to the table surface, then the angle in degrees between the thigh and the table represents the flexion contracture.

The knee is in a neutral position when the thigh and lower leg are in a straight line. If the knee extends past this neutral position, it is considered to be in hyperextension, also referred to as recurvatum. Flexion of the knee is determined by measuring the number of degrees between the thigh and lower leg when the knee is completely bent (Fig. 1-8). A flexion deformity of the knee (knee does not fully extend) is determined by measuring the number of degrees between the thigh and lower leg with the knee in maximum extension.

The ankle is in a neutral, or 0-degree, position when the foot is at a right angle to the leg. Dorsiflexion is measured when the entire foot is brought up toward the leg and the number of degrees between the foot and leg at the ankle joint is recorded. Plantar flexion is the motion of the foot at the ankle joint directed downwards or in an equinus position, and again the number of degrees between the leg and foot is recorded (Figs. 1-9, 1-10).

When describing the motion of the spine, the ability to bend forward is flexion, the ability to bend backward past the normal posture is extension, and the ability to bend to the right or left without flexing or extending is lateral bend.

The motion of the neck is described as follows: Flexion is bending the head forward; extension is moving the head backward; right lateral bending is moving the right ear to the right shoulder; left lateral bending is moving the left ear to the left shoulder; and rotation is turning the head from right to left or from left to right (Fig. 1-11).

In some instances, the nurse may measure limb circumference. In order for the measurements to be of value, the muscles must be relaxed, and the measurements should be performed at the same level on each side. This is accom-

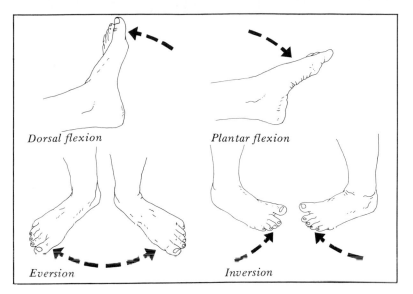

Dorsal flexion

Plantar flexion

Eversion

Inversion

Figure 1-9. Range of motion in the ankle and foot.

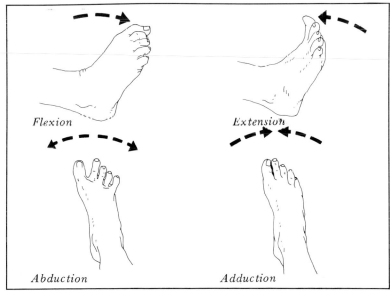

Flexion

Extension

Abduction

Adduction

Figure 1-10. Range of motion in the toe.

Figure 1-11. Range of motion in the neck.

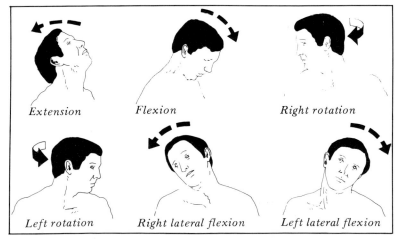

Extension

Flexion

Right rotation

Left rotation

Right lateral flexion

Left lateral flexion

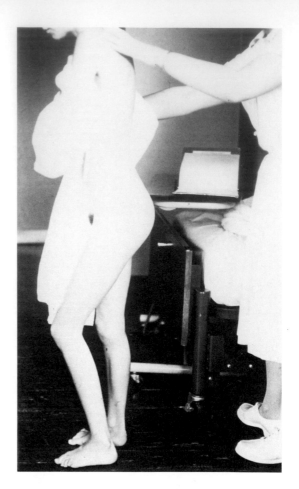

Figure 1-12. Short right leg secondary to congenital hip dislocation and growth abnormality. Note that the patient flexes the normal left knee to compensate.

plished by measuring an exact distance from a bony prominence on each limb and marking the location. The circumference of the limb is then measured at the skin mark with a tape measure.

Leg length discrepancies can affect the overall posture of an individual (Figs. 1-12, 1-13). Apparent leg lengths are measured from the umbilicus to the medial malleolus, the knees being straight up and the legs parallel. Positional changes in the hip can affect these measurements even when there is no true bony shortening or discrepancy. Real leg lengths are measured from the anterior superior iliac spine of the pelvis to the medial malleolus. Both legs should be measured in the same position. For example, if a patient has a stiff hip fixed in a position of abduction, the movable hip should be placed in the same position of abduction for measurement.

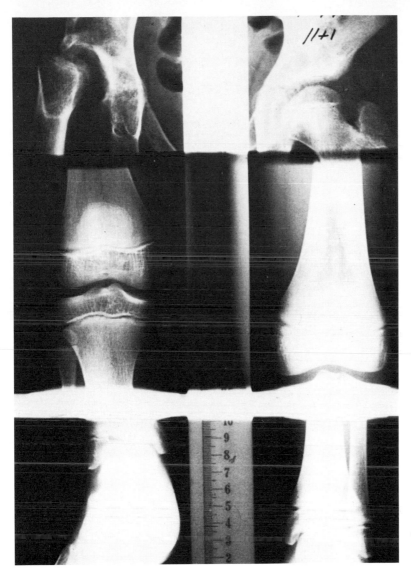

Figure 1-13. X-rays to document leg length discrepancy. This requires a special x-ray technique.

LABORATORY STUDIES

Although the nurse will not be ordering the diagnostic studies for the patient with a known or suspected orthopedic condition, it is desirable to have an understanding of them (Table 1-1). In order for the nursing assessment to be complete these reports should be reviewed and understood.

Some of the pertinent laboratory blood studies used frequently in orthopedics are: complete blood count; latex fixation, lupus erythematosus (LE) cell test, test for rheumatoid

*Table 1-1**

Serum Chemistries	Level	Disease/Condition
Serum calcium	Increased	Bone tumor (some cases) — acute osteo-porosis — multiple myeloma
	Decreased	Osteomalacia — rickets
Serum phosphorus	Increased	Healing fractures — multiple myeloma (some cases) — Paget's disease (some cases) — osteolytic metastatic tumor in bone (some cases) — acromegaly
	Decreased	Rickets — osteomalacia
Serum alkaline phosphatase	Increased	Paget's disease — healing fractures — osteoblastic bone tumors (osteogenic sarcoma, metastatic carcinoma) — osteogenesis imperfecta — osteomalacia — rickets — polyostotic fibrous dysplasia
Serum acid phosphatase	Increased	Paget's disease — metastatic prostatic carcinoma of bone — Gaucher's disease
Serum protein electro-phoresis	Increased protein	Multiple myeloma
	Decreased albumin	Multiple myeloma — rheumatoid arthritis — osteomyelitis
Serum uric acid	Increased	Gout
	Decreased	Use of uricosuric drugs (salicylates, cortisone, etc.) — acromegaly
Serum glucose	May be decreased	Fibrosarcoma
Serum urea nitrogen	May be decreased	Acromegaly
Serum creatinine	Increased	Gigantism — acromegaly — corticosteroid therapy
Serum creatine	Increased	Active rheumatoid arthritis — destruction of muscle
Serum cholesterol	Decreased	Cortisone therapy
Serum transaminase (SGOT)	Increased	Musculoskeletal disease — falsely increased with Prostaphlin, Polycillin, opiates, and Erythromycin therapy
Serum lactic dehydro-genase (LDH)	Increased	Pulmonary embolism infarction (complication frequently seen in orthopedic nursing)
Serum alpha — hydroxy-butyric dehydrogenase (alpha — HBD)	Increased	Muscular dystrophy
Serum creatine phospha-kinase (CPK)	Increased	Progressive muscular dystrophy — poly-myositis — traumatic injury of muscle (increase may last 10–14 days, particularly if associated with arterial obstruction)
Serum globulins	Increased	Rheumatoid arthritis (beta 2M) — multiple myeloma (beta 2A)
Serum C — reactive protein	Not normally detected in serum	
	Increased	Any acute inflammatory change or necrosis — widespread metastasis — rheumatoid arthritis

*Adapted from Jacques Wallach, *Interpretation of Diagnostic Tests* (2nd ed.). Boston: Little Brown, 1974.

factor, and antistreptococcal antibody titers (ASOT), all tests for rheumatoid arthritis; erythrocyte sedimentation rate, which is elevated in rheumatoid arthritis, pyogenic arthritis, myeloma, and infections; blood coagulation studies, used not only for diagnosis and to determine baselines, but also to determine therapeutic levels for drug administration; serum salicylate level; and serum chemistries (Table 1-1).

The following urinalysis results are also pertinent to orthopedics: Urine calcium may be increased in lytic bone lesions (metastatic tumor, multiple myeloma); it is decreased in rickets, osteomalacia, and metastatic carcinoma of the prostate. There is an increased formation of urine creatine in muscle dystrophy, myasthenia gravis, crush injury, acromegaly, and drug therapy with adrenocorticotropic hormone (ACTH) and cortisone; an increased breakdown of urine creatine is present with infections, burns, and fractures. Bence Jones proteinuria is usually diagnostic of multiple myeloma, as is a positive urinary electrophoretic pattern.

Synovial (joint) fluid may be examined grossly and microscopically to differentiate acute inflammatory arthritis of various etiologies.

X-RAY INTERPRETATION

X-rays are the most frequently used diagnostic tool in orthopedics today. The review of x-rays and x-ray reports is an important part of the assessment of the orthopedic patient.

An orthopedic nurse should be familiar with the normal as well as the abnormal of x ray interpretation. It is desirable to have some basic knowledge in interpretation of orthopedic x-rays. This ability enables the nurse to more reasonably plan and participate in the care of the orthopedic patient.

X-rays are made in order to gain more information in evaluating an individual's problem. An x-ray of the bone and soft tissues may give information that can lead to the diagnosis of a patient's difficulty, whether it be a fracture, bone tumor, bone disease, abnormality of development, calcification in a bursa, or swelling of soft tissues.

In general, x-rays can best be thought of as shadows of structures, particularly bony structures. A simple and effective way to gain a better understanding of what x-rays show is to hold a pencil up behind or in front of a light at night and see how the light and the pencil cast a shadow on the wall (Fig. 1-14). This is exactly what one sees when looking at an x-ray. A shadow of the bone is cast on the x-ray film due to the fact that the bone blocks the x-ray beam going through the tissues, just as the pencil blocks the light. Bones are denser than other tissues and do not allow the x-ray beams to

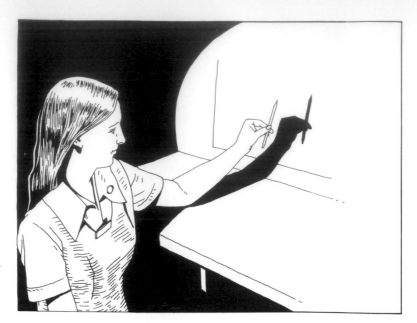

Figure 1-14. Note shadow of hand and pencil on wall.

Figure 1-15. An- teroposterior (top) and lateral (bottom) views of the knee.

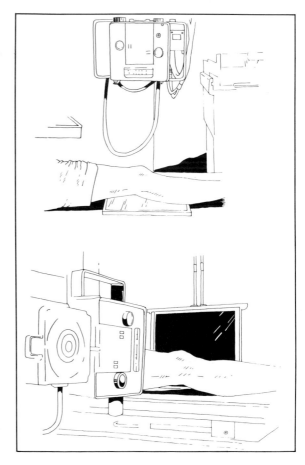

penetrate them; wherever this density occurs, the x-ray film develops white.

It must be understood that x-rays are not three-dimensional, and therefore do not indicate depth. Often, to identify the relationships of the structures studied one must look at them in two planes at 90-degree angles to each other; furthermore, oblique x-rays may be needed to clarify these structures.

The most frequent views used are the anteroposterior (AP), lateral, and oblique views. In an AP view, the x-ray is made with the tube facing the front of the structure and the x-ray is made from front to back. In a similar manner, a posteroanterior (PA) view is made with the tube facing the back of the structure and the x-ray is then made from back to front. The resultant x-ray is the same, but for convenience most often the AP view will be made. For a lateral view the x-ray tube faces the structure from the side, and when an oblique view is made the x-ray tube faces the structure from an angle (Fig. 1-15).

Anteroposterior and lateral views are almost always needed. For example, an internal fixation device for the fixation of a hip fracture could actually be placed on the skin in front of the hip, and on an AP x-ray the film would show perfect posi-

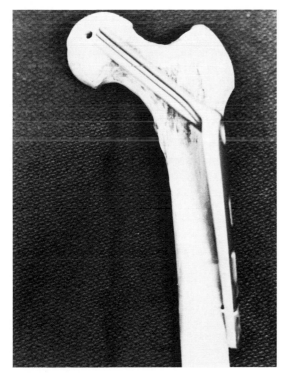

Figure 1-16. Fixation device placed in front of the hip.

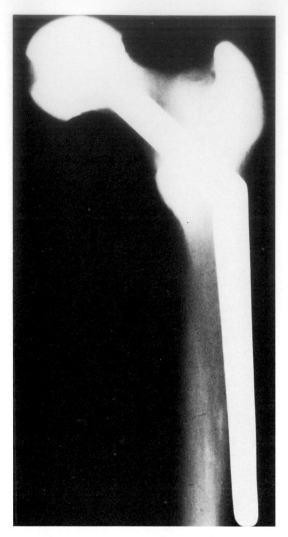

Figure 1-17. The anteroposterior x-ray of Figure 1-16 looks perfect.

tion of the device in the head and neck of the femur (Figs. 1-16, 1-17). When a lateral x-ray of this is made, the nail is shown to be in front of the hip, not in the bone (Figs. 1-18, 1-19). In determining the position of a fracture, it is necessary to have these two views and occasionally an oblique view. Frequently an AP view of a fracture will show it to be in good position whereas the lateral or oblique view will show it to be offset or displaced.

Special views are occasionally necessary for adequate examination. A lateral x-ray of the cervical spine may be made in flexion and extension to determine whether changes in position cause any abnormal subluxation. A fracture in the wrist

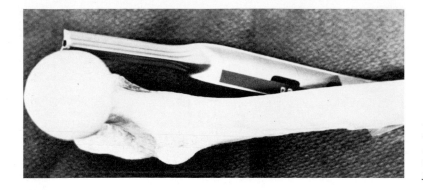

Figure 1-18. Lateral view of the hip with the fixation device in front.

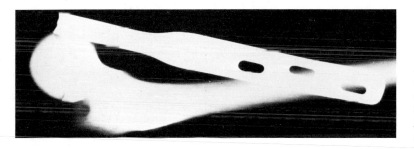

Figure 1-19. Lateral x-ray clearly shows the fixation device in front of the hip (see Fig. 1-18).

navicular is often not seen on standard views, but may be detected on special views.

The various x-ray views may be more understandable through the following simple experiment. The materials needed are a piece of wire bent into an S shape and a desk light. Allow the light to throw a shadow of the wire on the wall, and slowly rotate the wire. Any rotation between 0 and 90 degrees can vary the shadow shown. If this same piece of wire is laid flat on a x-ray cassette and an x-ray is made with the tube facing the wire in a straight line, an S is seen on the developed film. However, if the wire is held on its side or edge and a x-ray is made with the tube in the same position, the wire appears on the film as a straight line (Fig. 1-20). This experiment demonstrates not only the necessity for different views but also why there is a limitation in the interpretation of x-rays.

X-ray film should be placed on a viewbox for viewing. In general, viewing an anteroposterior x-ray is just like looking at the front of a skeleton. Thus, when an AP x-ray of a pelvis is placed on the viewbox the right hip will be to one's left (Fig. 1-21); an AP x-ray of the tibias should be placed so that the fibulas are to the outside. X-rays of the hand and wrist or of the forearm including the wrist should

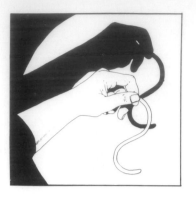
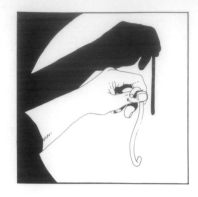

Figure 1-20. Note how projection of S changes with rotation.

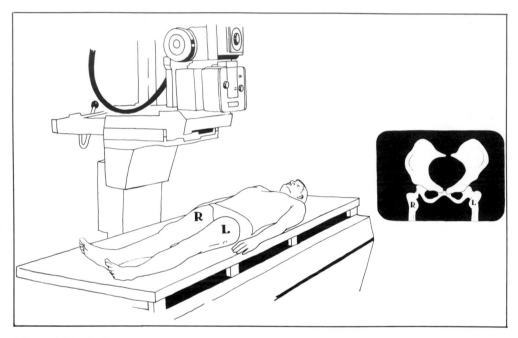

Figure 1-21. Technique of making an anteroposterior x-ray of the pelvis and proper positioning on the viewbox.

be placed with the fingers up. Conversely, x-rays of the forearm with the elbow should be placed with the elbow facing up and the forearm down. X-rays of the toes and feet should be placed with the toes up; x-rays of the ankle should be placed as if one is looking at the patient. These same guidelines may be followed for other x-rays; always place the x-ray film as if one is looking at the patient, with the patient's right side to the examiner's left. An exception to this is made when viewing scoliosis x-rays. The films are usually anteroposterior, but they are placed on the viewbox as if the x-ray tube was

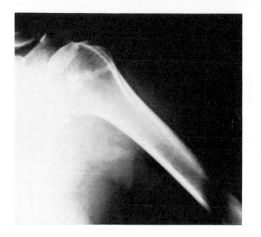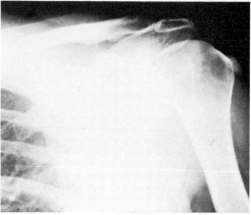

Figure 1-22. Note calcium in soft tissue just lateral to the head of the left humerus in this patient with calcific bursitis.

behind the patient. The patient's right side on the film will be to the viewer's right.

X-ray interpretation is complex; however, there are basic guidelines to follow. When viewing an x-ray observe all of the following: *surrounding soft tissues; contours of the bone; periosteal reaction and callus; bone destruction; and general density of the bone.*

The *surrounding soft tissue* should be scrutinized for calcification such as is seen in calcific bursitis, tendinitis, or any ectopic bone formation (Fig. 1-22). Unusual shadows should also be noted; these may indicate gas in the tissues from a penetrating wound or gas gangrene. Swelling in the tissues suggests recent injury, the presence of fluid, inflammation, or a soft tissue tumor.

When viewing the *contours of the bone* one should find the overall shape to be normal; the cartilage will not usually show up on an x-ray but will appear as radiolucent space. The epiphysis should be noted when present but epiphyseal development and contour may normally vary from individual to individual (Fig. 1-23); the best and the most instructive guide to what is normal is a comparison with an x-ray of the uninvolved side. When the contour of the bone is altered from normal this change may be due to a break in the cortex of the bone by a fracture or an outgrowth of the bone such as an osteochondroma, arthritic osteophyte, or other abnormal condition. It may also be due to arthritis, which will cause irregular contours adjacent to joints. Narrowing of the joint space is caused by arthritis. A fracture may be detected by observing a break in continuity around the edge of the bone or a radio-

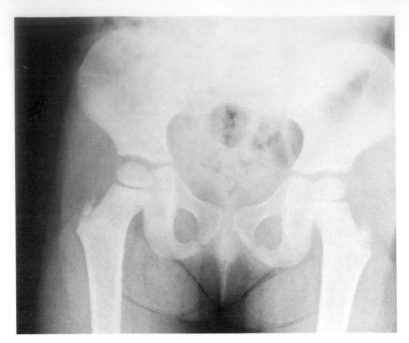

Figure 1-23. Anteroposterior x-ray of the pelvis in a child. Note joint space (cartilage) in each hip and the normal epiphyseal lines in both hips.

lucent line across the substance of the bone; fresh fracture lines are usually sharp and distinct, whereas normal vascular channels are round and smooth (Fig. 1-24).

Periosteal cells respond to injury by forming new bone (callus). If new bone formation from the periosteum is seen, it may be a normal healing response to a fracture or it can mean that the periosteum has been traumatized by a direct blow or tumor growth. Periosteal healing may identify a fracture that was not seen on the initial x-rays; sharp radiolucent lines of a fresh fracture become fuzzy and smoother as bone healing occurs. Observation for *periosteal reaction* and *callus* should always be included when viewing an x-ray film.

Bone destruction has a variety of forms. Acute infection (osteomyelitis) and certain malignant bone tumors cause a moth-eaten appearance of the bone, which represents a form of bone destruction (Fig. 1-25). Advanced arthritic conditions may result in destruction of the subchondral bone. Smooth-bordered radiolucent shadows are cystic benign lesions (Fig. 1-26). Metastatic lesions (especially from sites in the kidney and thyroid) may appear on the x-ray as punched-out areas in the bone. Some metastatic lesions, however, espe-

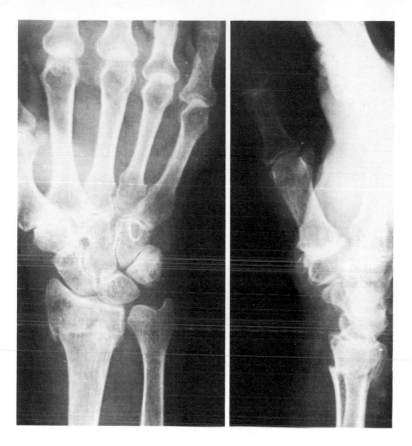

Figure 1-24. Anteroposterior and lateral x-rays of the wrist. Note fracture line in the distal radius (Colles' fracture).

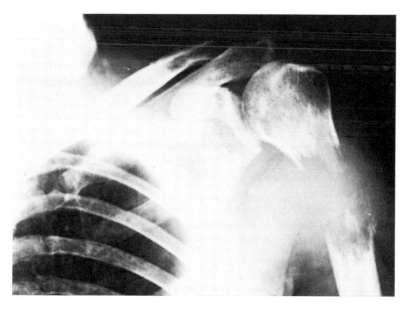

Figure 1-25. Metastatic carcinoma of the left humerus causing bone destruction.

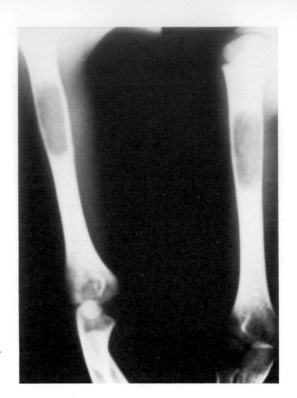

Figure 1-26. Bone cyst in the right humerus.

cially from the breast and prostate, may evoke an osteoblastic reaction.

The *general density of the bone* must also be considered when viewing an x-ray. A *decrease* in density of the bone may be due to several factors: increased circulation to the bone from any type of inflammatory disease, such as rheumatoid arthritis; circulatory abnormalities, such as arteriovenous fistulas and hemangiomas; and infection. Normal stress is necessary for new bone formation and calcium deposition in the new bone. When there is decreased use of a limb, over a period of time there will actually be less protein and less calcium salts in that extremity (disuse osteoporosis); the x-ray will manifest this by actually looking less white, or less dense. In osteoporosis in older people this same principle is operating, as are hormonal factors that may influence its development.

An *increase* in the density (sclerosis) of the bone should be recognized when viewing any x-ray film. New bone formation, such as is seen in healing fractures, causes an increase in density; it is important to know that some areas normally form more callus than others when a fracture heals. Decreased bone resorption also causes an increase in density.

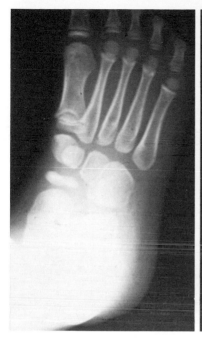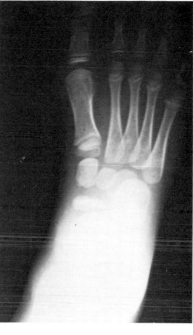

Figure 1-27. Aseptic necrosis of the tarsal navicular (scaphoid).

This condition is seen in cases of sequestrum (dead bone from an infection with no blood supply) and in aseptic necrosis where the blood supply has been interrupted (Fig. 1-27). Other conditions which are manifested as an increase in density are osteogenic primary bone tumors, metastatic lesions that evoke an osteoblastic response (such as those from the breast and prostate), and Paget's disease. In arthritis the body's normal repair response to the arthritic process may increase local bone production, producing sclerosis.

Standard x-rays are frequently ordered, as are other diagnostic studies, to rule out bony involvement. This is particularly true in patients with back pain or knee injuries. Disc and cartilage are not visible on x-rays; although the clinical findings indicate a disc or cartilage abnormality, it is important to rule out any involvement of bone by x-ray.

Since cartilage and disc are not visible on standard x-rays, special x-ray procedures are often required to obtain more information concerning these structures.

A *discogram* is a special x-ray procedure that provides more information concerning the condition of a disc. It is done by placing a needle in the disc space and injecting a contrast medium that is radiopaque. This procedure is relatively difficult to perform and interpret; therefore, it is not a valuable study for many orthopedic surgeons.

A much more valuable and widely used diagnostic tool in

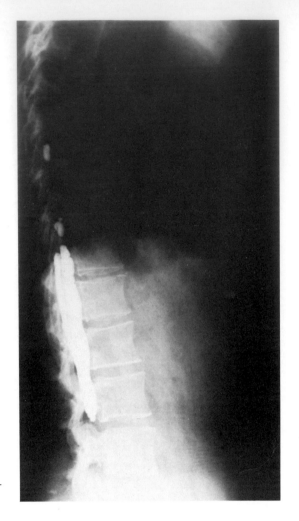

Figure 1-28. My-elogram.

evaluating disc problems is the *myelogram* (Fig. 1-28). A myelogram is performed by placing a needle in the subarachnoid space of the spine (as in a spinal tap) and inserting a radiopaque contrast medium into this area. This contrast medium is then visualized by fluoroscopy as it flows up and down the spinal subarachnoid space. If a disc is protruding significantly posteriorly, the contrast medium will be pushed to the side. This displacement of the medium can be caused by any space-occupying lesion, such as a herniated disc or nerve root tumor. As in all other findings, the clinical findings together with the x-rays will provide the data for a final diagnosis.

Arthrograms are x-rays that give information pertaining to the shape and outline of the cartilaginous surfaces of a joint (Fig. 1-29). A needle is inserted into the major joint to be

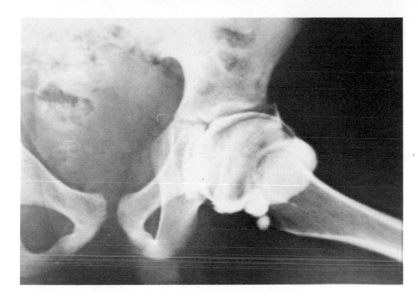

Figure 1-29. Arthrogram.

visualized, and radiopaque contrast medium is injected. This medium outlines the surfaces of the joint. An arthrogram may also be used to determine the integrity of the capsule of a joint.

Tomograms are x-rays made at different levels of a structure and are usually performed by a radiologist (Fig. 1-30). This technique is used when standard x-rays would not disclose the lesion or when the appearance of the lesion is less than adequate. For example, an osteoid-osteoma is a small solitary lesion, usually less than 2 cm in diameter, found in the cortex of a bone and difficult to identify on standard x-rays. With the use of tomography a more definite location may be determined by making an x-ray of the bone at different levels.

Bone scanning is another diagnostic x-ray study. It is used primarily for the detection of bone metastases; however, due to new advances which have decreased time and cost, it is now being used for evaluation of benign disease. Generally the bone scan identifies those areas in which there is any increased bone activity or active bone formation (fracture, infection, and others). When reading a bone scan, the normal bone deposition is usually recorded as dark gray photodots and the abnormalities appear as black areas on a gray background. This study is performed after an injection of radioactive isotopes.

A diagnostic study of the bone that is done in conjunction with x-ray is the Craig needle biopsy. This procedure is a closed biopsy of the bone using a special needle. Localization

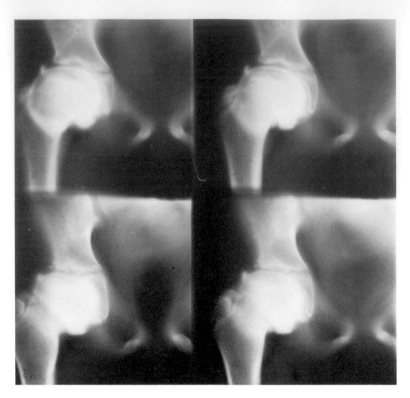

Figure 1-30.
Tomograms.

of the needle (trocar) in the suspected lesion is assured through the use of standard x-rays or fluoroscopy.

Nursing assessment, like all other steps of the nursing process, must be done concurrently and recurrently.

NURSING DIAGNOSIS

The summary statement(s) of the nursing assessment is the nursing diagnosis. The term *nursing diagnosis* has been considered by many to be controversial; however, when used appropriately it is the summation of the nursing assessment. Presenting problems must be identified in order to establish goals and a plan of nursing care for any orthopedic patient.

A nursing diagnosis, the establishment of goals, and a plan of nursing care all must be based on an understanding of the common disease processes or conditions that affect the normal function of the musculoskeletal system and their anticipated course, as well as the accepted clinical management of these problems.

SUGGESTED READINGS

Abdellah, F.G., et al.: *Patient-Centered Approaches to Nursing.* New York: Macmillan, 1960.

Ackerman, Susan: The orthopedic nursing diagnosis. *Orthop. Nurs. Assoc. J.* 2:58–59, March 1975.

Ackerman, Susan: Orthopedic nurses make thorough assessment of orthopedic patients. *Orthop. Nurs. Assoc. J.* 2:108–109, May 1975.

Bloch, Doris: Some crucial terms in nursing: What do they really mean? *Nurs. Outlook* 22:689–694, 1974.

Bower, F.L.: The process of planning nursing care: a theoretical model. *Nurs. Outlook* 22:85, 1974.

Burrill, Marjorie: Helping students identify and solve patients' problems. *Nurs. Outlook* 14:46–48, 1966.

Carrieri, V.K., et al.: Components of the nursing process. *Nurs. Clin. North Am.* 6:115–124, 1971.

Gebbie, K., and Lavin, M. A. : Classifying nursing diagnoses. *Am. J. Nurs.* 74:250–253. 1974.

Kelly, N.C.: Nursing Care Plans. *Nurs. Outlook* 14:61–63, 1966.

Little, D.E., and Carnevali, D.L.: *Nursing Care Planning*. Philadelphia: J.B. Lippincott, 1969.

McCain, R.F.: Nursing by assessment—not intuition. *Am. J. Nurs.* 65:82–84, 1965.

May, Eleanor A., and Sells, Clifford J.: Scoliosis screening in public schools. *Am. J. Nurs.* 74:60–62, 1974.

Mayers, Marlene Glover: *A Systematic Approach to the Nursing Care Plan*. New York: Meredith Corp., 1972.

Nowlin, Ouida: Guidelines for pediatric orthopedic nursing history. *Orthop. Nurs. Assoc. J.* 2:119, May 1975.

Orlando, Ida Jean: *The Discipline and Teaching of Nursing Process* (An Evaluative Study). New York: Putnam, 1972.

Schubert, Wanda, and Gunn, Norma: Adapting nursing histories for orthopedics. *Orthop. Nurs. Assoc. J.* 1:96–97, November 1974.

Wagner, B.M.: Care plans: right, reasonable, and reachable. *Am. J. Nurs.* 69:986–990, 1969.

Yura, Helen, and Walsh, Mary B.: *The Nursing Process: Assessing, Planning, Implementing and Evaluating* (2nd ed.). New York: Meredith Corp., 1973.

2. TRAUMA

INITIAL NURSING ASSESSMENT

In any injury or emergency, everyone's attention is immediately directed to the local site of the obvious injury. The overall assessment must include evaluation not only of the obvious injury, but also of the patient's general status. This must be accomplished quickly, but thoroughly, before proceeding with any nursing actions concerning the obvious injury. The patient's airway breathing, and bleeding must be evaluated. The physical assessment must always include observation for signs and symptoms of a head, chest, or abdominal injury. Remember, an open fracture of the femur may appear to be the most serious injury, but in many instances may in fact not be the most urgent. With normal findings referable to these areas on the initial assessment, appropriate attention can then be directed to the local problem.

An assessment of the injury must include a neurovascular check of the area distal to the injury. A complete neurovascular check must include evaluation of the following: capillary filling, color, temperature, edema, pulses, sensory nerve function, and motor nerve function.

Remember, an injury sufficient to fracture a long extremity bone or dislocate a joint may also cause fracture at a higher level, dislocation of a proximal joint, or both. An adequate assessment of the entire extremity is imperative.

INITIAL NURSING ACTIONS

All wounds should have sterile dressings applied to them as soon as possible, thereby decreasing the chance of infection. Any bleeding should be controlled by applying pressure over the sterile dressing manually or with an elastic bandage wrap over a bulky sterile dressing.

All fractures should be splinted. A pillow splint may be used for the foot, ankle, tibia, and knee. For a fractured femur, a Thomas splint with traction or a modification thereof should be applied. Often, simply adjusting the leg in a position of comfort on a pillow is satisfactory for temporary splinting and management of the fractured hip; be sure the pillow elevates the heel and ankle off the bed to avoid development of pressure areas. A fractured hip is frequently placed in Buck's traction as a comfort measure. Frequently the most effective way to splint a forearm or elbow fracture is to have the patient cradle the arm in the uninjured arm (if the patient is calm and cooperative). Splinting of fractures or injuries of the shoulder and humeral shaft is often accomplished by a simple stockinette sling around the neck and wrist, which allows the weight of the suspended arm to align the fracture and thus gives temporary splinting, with the patient in a sitting or semisitting position. Contour plaster splints may be used effectively in an emergency room. Approximately 8 to 10 thicknesses of plaster are cut to the appropriate length and width. After the plaster has been dipped in water and backed with sheet cotton, Webril, or Sofrol, it is gently applied to the extremity in its position of deformity (as it is) and carefully wrapped in place with a gauze or elastic bandage wrap. Although the splint may obscure some details of an x-ray, this drawback is more than compensated for by the relief of pain and protection of the extremity from further injury that might be caused by unnecessary motion.

Control of pain is accomplished through immobilization by appropriate splinting, judicious use of narcotics, and much reassurance to the patient. Maintenance of blood pressure is enhanced by adequate control of pain. Rapid changes in position should always be avoided.

Orthostatic hypotension can be avoided by encouraging the patient to move the feet and ankles while sitting. Do not have a patient sit on the examining table without adequate assistance with the legs in a dependent position for evaluation and treatment of an injury such as a fracture of the clavicle or shoulder.

There must be preparation for thorough cleansing and débridement of damaged and nonviable tissue. Cleanly incised wounds require only irrigation and closure, whereas crush injuries require wide open débridement and inspection, sometimes with delayed or secondary closure.

FRACTURES AND JOINT INJURIES
Fractures
It must be remembered that bone is a living tissue that absorbs normal stresses and strains. A fracture is an abnormal break in the usual continuity of a bone. When such a break occurs, not only is there damage and death of some of the living cells of the bone, but there also is injury to the covering of the bone, the periosteum, as well as to surrounding tissues.

When a bone is broken, bleeding from damaged blood vessels causes the formation of a hematoma at the fracture site. This hematoma is gradually invaded by capillaries and fibrous tissue. A metaplastic process occurs and callus, or fibrocartilage, is formed by the body. This is gradually transformed into bone, with reestablishment of continuity and strength of the bone across the fracture site. This process occurs to a greater extent around the outside of a long bone (periosteal healing) (Fig. 2-1) and to a lesser extent in the intramedullary

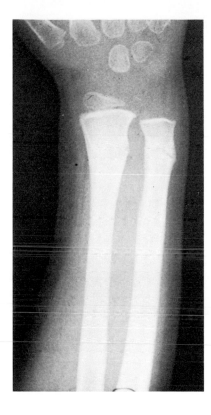

Figure 2-1. Heal-ing fractures of the distal radius and ulna. Note the periosteal healing.

canal (endosteal healing). Certain bones and locations tend to show more or less exuberant healing callus than others.

Because of the break in the continuity of the bone, as well as damage to the adjacent nerves, blood vessels, muscles, and other soft tissues, the occurrence of a fracture causes pain. Deformity may or may not be present. The patient may be able to move the involved extremity even after a fracture, depending on the stability of the fracture.

It is helpful to use the terms *open*, for fractures in which the skin over the fracture is open (Fig. 2-2), and *closed*, for fractures in which the continuity of the skin overlying the fracture is not interrupted (Fig. 2-3). *Open* and *closed* are more meaningful terms than *simple* and *compound*. For example, a fracture can be very complex and difficult to manage even though the skin is intact, and certainly should not be considered a simple fracture. The term *compound* can often be confused with the terms *complex* and *comminuted*; therefore, to avoid misunderstanding it is best to call all fractures in which the skin is opened, open fractures (Fig. 2-4). The other terms can then be applied as descriptions of the actual fracture site. The term *comminuted* describes a fracture with several pieces (Fig. 2-5). *Greenstick, buckle,* and *torus* are used to de-

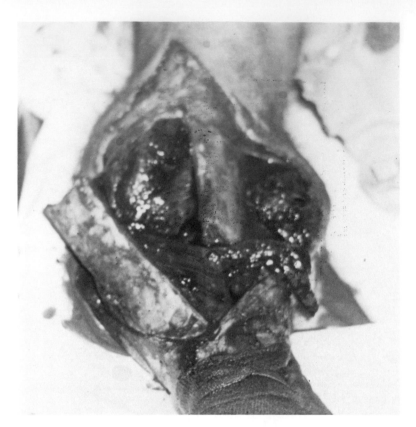

Figure 2-2. Open fracture of the tibia and fibula.

Figure 2-3. Closed fracture-disloca-tion of the left hip.

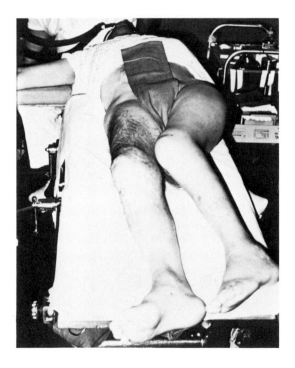

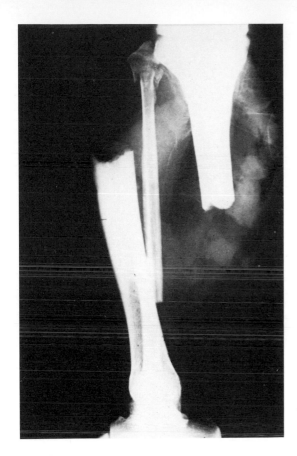

Figure 2-4. X-ray of an open fracture of the tibia and fibula.

scribe a fracture in which there is simply a crimp in the bone, with the periosteum maintaining an overall continuity.

A *fracture-separation* of the *epiphysis* is a type of fracture in which the line of discontinuity of the bone occurs at the cartilaginous epiphyseal line at the ends of the long bones (Fig. 2-6).

Pathological fractures are fractures occurring in an area of the bone that withstands stress less well than normal due to some process already occurring in the bone which weakens it (Fig. 2-7). For example, the young adolescent who draws an arm back to throw a pass sustains a pathological fracture when the humerus fractures through a previous bone cyst.

Occasionally, prolonged stress applied at one area of the bone will cause an undisplaced fracture of the bone, with pain on weight bearing. This is called a stress fracture. An x-ray made shortly after this fracture occurs will be normal. However, as the stress fracture gradually heals, a radiolucent line with a nearby increased density and sclerosis is seen. The periosteum will often be elevated in the area, with some new

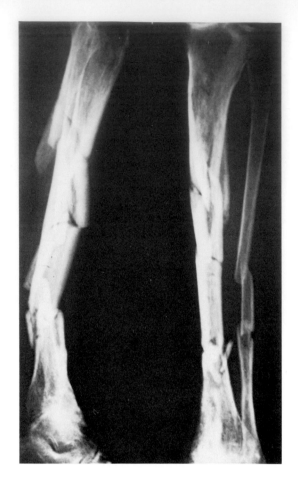

Figure 2-5. X-ray of a comminuted fracture of the tibia and fibula.

bone formation; this indicates the healing of the stress fracture (Fig. 2-8).

Fractures may occur as the result of direct or indirect stresses on the bone. Direct trauma is stress applied directly to the bone through the soft tissues overlying it. Indirect stress is torsion (torque) applied to the bone by forces initially acting on the body or extremity at some distance from the fracture site: for example, in a skier, when the ski catches in the snow and torque is applied to the foot and ankle in the ski boot, the combination of forces often causes the tibia and fibula to fracture above the ankle and foot.

COMPLICATIONS OF FRACTURES. The orthopedic nurse should be familiar with the complications of fractures. Those associated with union are classified as malunion, delayed union, and nonunion.

When the fractured bone is healed, but is in a position that does not allow satisfactory function, this is classified as a *mal-*

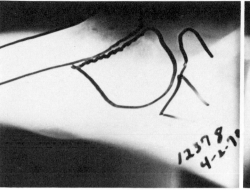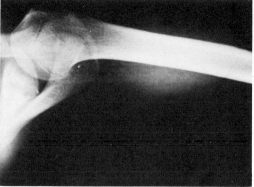

Figure 2-6. Frac-
ture-separation of
the proximal hu-
meral epiphysis,
showing unaf-
fected shoulder
for comparison.

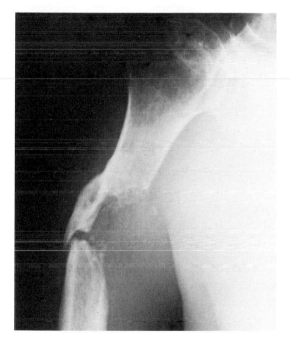

Figure 2-7. Path-
ological fracture
of the right hu-
merus.

union (Fig. 2-9). This complication may be treated by an
osteotomy to correct the alignment (Fig. 2-10).

Delayed union occurs when a fracture heals much more
slowly than one would normally expect. If after a prolonged
period of time no bony union occurs, it is then called a nonunion, and at this time it is not usually anticipated that healing will occur without some type of intervention to stimulate
it. A nonunion is usually treated by some type of bone graft-

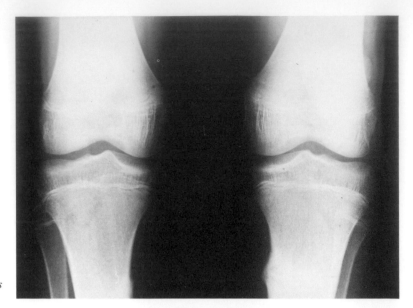

Figure 2-8. Healing stress fractures of both tibias.

Figure 2-9. Malunion of the right tibia preoperatively.

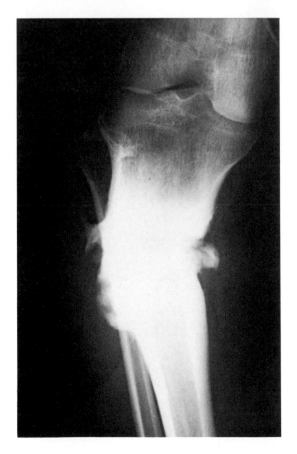

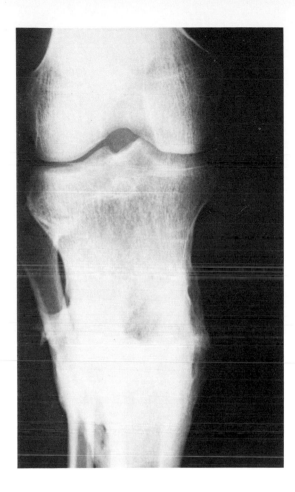

Figure 2-10. Mal-union of the right tibia after osteot-omy and correc-tion.

ing procedure to stimulate healing across the fracture site. An autogenous cancellous-bone graft from the ilium or a sliding cortical-bone graft from the adjacent bone or ilium is used. Internal fixation may or may not be utilized along with the bone grafting procedure.

Complications may also occur in surrounding soft tissues. Skin necrosis can occur over fractures (Fig. 2-11). It occurs most often in areas of relatively poor circulation (particularly over the anterior aspect of the tibia) where underlying swelling causes tenseness and tightness in the skin, leading to capillary compression and anoxia of the skin tissues. This can also occur when the fracture angulates, pressing the skin against the bone and cast and causing anoxia of the skin tissues and tissue death.

When muscle is traumatized, bruised, and hemorrhagic, a condition called myositis ossificans can occur (Fig. 2-12). This poorly understood condition is characterized by the formation of new bone in the muscular area adjacent to the under-

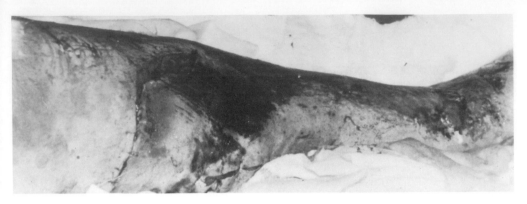

*Figure 2-11. Skin
necrosis after se-
vere open frac-
ture.*

*Figure 2-12. My-
ositis ossificans of
the quadriceps.*

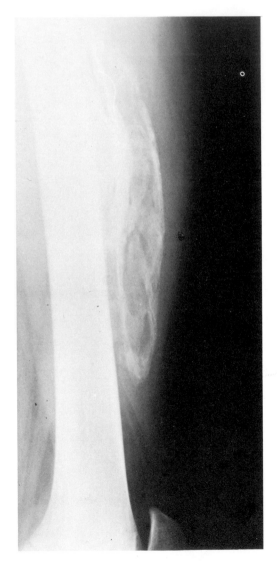

lying bone, and can result in limitation of motion of the extremity. Operative excision of an area of myositis ossificans while it is going through its developing and maturing stage usually results in more myositis ossificans; for this reason excision, when necessary, is delayed until the new bone has completely matured.

Tendons and muscles can occasionally become embedded in scar in an area of a healing fracture. This can result in severance of the tendon with use or in limitation in the range of motion of a muscle, its tendon, or both, and can thereby limit the motion of the adjacent joints.

Nerves and blood vessels can become damaged by the ends of a fracture or entrapped in fracture callus, causing neurovascular dysfunction.

Occasionally *Sudeck's atrophy*, a little understood reflex sympathetic dystrophy, occurs. This complication is not necessarily related to the degree of trauma. Occasionally, after an injury such as a Colles' fracture of the wrist or even a simple undisplaced fracture of the ankle, a patient will have an edematous, cool, and sensitive extremity, with pain on attempted use and weight bearing, which resists all forms of physical therapy and pain relief. The bone involved often shows marked osteopenia, more so than one would expect from the disuse (Fig. 2-13). Treatment is difficult and usually involves spending a lot of time encouraging the individual to gradually use the extremity. Sympathetic nerve blocks may have a part in treatment.

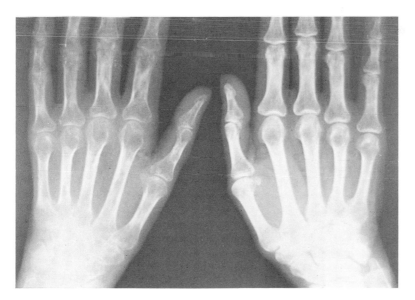

Figure 2-13. Osteoporosis of the left hand secondary to Sudeck's atrophy.

General Principles of Fracture Treatment

The general principles involved in the treatment of fractures are centered around restoration of the individual with a fracture to normal function, if possible. In the treatment of a fracture, the surrounding soft tissues, including the skin, nerves, muscles, and vascular system, must always be considered. A beautifully aligned bone as seen on an x-ray, with healing, is of little use to a patient if in the treatment process nerve and vascular functions are lost and the limb is atrophic and does not function.

Fortunately, most fractures can be treated by the closed method. Children's fractures can be treated successfully by closed means more often than fractures in adults, because children's bones have a great capacity to remodel offset and angulation in the plane of the function of a joint (Fig. 2-14). Children also have a much tougher, thicker periosteum than adults; therefore, one sees fewer severely displaced fractures in children than in adults.

Any operation on a bone damages its adjacent structures and soft tissues. Nevertheless, in certain cases problems of restoring the patient to function and maintaining the fractured bone in an acceptable, functional position necessitate open treatment. In every case the advantages are weighed against the disadvantages and action is taken accordingly.

Open reduction of a fracture means the skin is opened and the fracture is exposed in order to reduce it so that acceptable position and alignment are obtained. Fractures that gener-

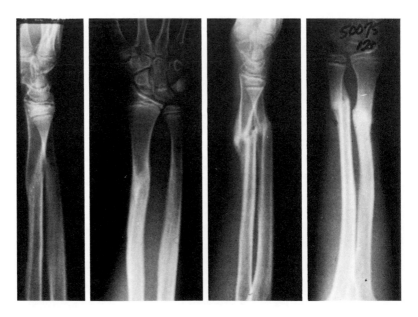

Figure 2-14. Note remodeling of this arm fracture over a six-month period.

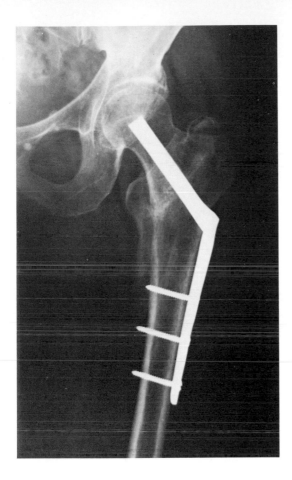

Figure 2-15. Open reduction and internal fixation of an intertrochanteric fracture of the left hip.

ally are better treated by open reduction and internal fixation, as opposed to closed methods, are hip fractures (Fig. 2-15), displaced fractures of the forearm in adults (Fig. 2-16), and displaced fractures of the ankle in adults (Fig. 2-17). Certain other fractures are often treated by open reduction and internal fixation; in every case it is a matter of the orthopedic surgeon's judgment as to the relative risks and advantages of open as opposed to closed treatment.

Fractures can be immobilized by external means, including slings, casts, and splints, or by internal means such as plates, nails, pins, wires, and other devices.

Joint Injuries

If the two bones that make up the joint are completely separated and no longer articulate, then a *dislocation* has occurred. This implies a rupture of the joint capsule and synovium, as well as a certain amount of trauma to the adjacent muscles and soft tissues. In a *subluxation,* the two articular surfaces

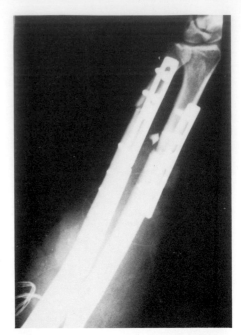

Figure 2-16. Open reduction and internal fixation of a fracture of both bones of the forearm.

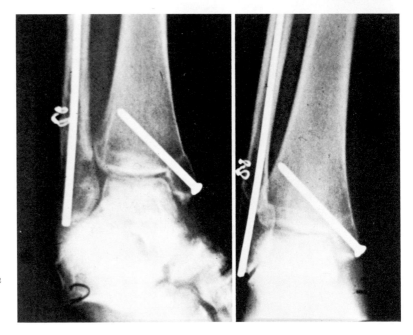

Figure 2-17. Open reduction and internal fixation of an ankle fracture.

that make up the joint are not entirely congruous, but are at least partially articulating. A subluxation similarly implies a stretching and loosening of the joints, synovium, and capsule, although not necessarily a complete rupture of the capsule.

A dislocation of a joint is a surgical emergency because the increased swelling and edema that occur when the joint is dislocated can damage soft tissues and cause changes in the capsule, ligaments, and muscles about the involved joint, preventing easy reduction. The facility of reduction of a dislocation varies inversely with the time after the injury at which reduction is attempted. Similarly, damage to muscles, blood vessels, nerves, and tendons around a dislocated joint increases in direct proportion to the length of time the reduction is delayed.

Following reduction of a dislocation, the joint is immobilized or placed at rest in order to make the patient more comfortable, allow the swollen and damaged adjacent soft tissues to return to their normal state, and permit the capsule and lining of the joint to heal. In general, 3 to 6 weeks of protection and immobilization of some sort are necessary following most initial joint dislocations.

Just as important as appropriate immobilization to allow healing of soft tissues around the joint is mobilization to restore range of motion and normal function of the muscles and tissues that surround the joint. In general, after most dislocations gradual, gentle range of motion exercises are begun at some time between 3 and 6 weeks after the dislocation is reduced. Setting exercises with the joint in the stable position of reduction can begin as soon as comfort permits.

Other joint injuries are *sprain*, which refers to stretching of the ligaments surrounding a joint but not a complete tear of the ligaments, and *strain*, which refers to stretching of the muscles.

A dislocation of the joint with an associated fracture of one or both of the bones comprising the joint is referred to as a fracture-dislocation (Fig. 2-18).

Rehabilitation of Fractures and Joint Injuries
When one expects normal function to return in an injured area, rehabilitation involves guiding it gently and progressively on its course of return to normal without delaying the healing process. Timing is of the utmost importance, since immobilization for too long a period often can result in irreversible changes in the capsule, muscles, and soft tissues about a joint, permanently limiting motion in the future. Conversely, too early mobilization can result in inadequate healing of the capsule and tissues about a joint, with permanent laxity and dysfunction. Rehabilitation, therefore, requires knowing not only how to restore function, but also when to encourage this restoration. When one anticipates significant remaining disability in spite of maximum efforts at rehabilitation, the rehabilitation effort, in addition to restoring to an individual

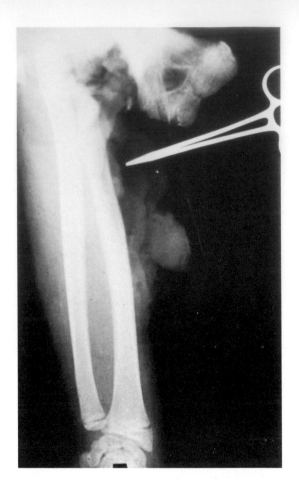

Figure 2-18. Fracture-dislocation of the elbow.

maximum possible function, also involves helping him or her to adjust to permanent limitations and assisting in obtaining the appropriate devices to facilitate function with this permanent disability. This involves psychological as well as physiological preparation.

Skeletal Injuries of the Trunk

The spinal cord and cauda equina are protected by the vertebral bodies that comprise the cervical, thoracic, and lumbar spine. Strong, tough ligaments and muscles stabilize the bony vertebrae and resist their displacement, thereby further protecting the essential spinal cord and its nerve roots. The consequences of injury to the vertebrae are related primarily to whether the spinal cord and nerves are damaged rather than to the injury to the skeletal system itself. For example, in a fracture of a vertebral body with no instability (danger of further displacement) or injury to the spinal cord and nerves, the treatment is primarily symptomatic until healing

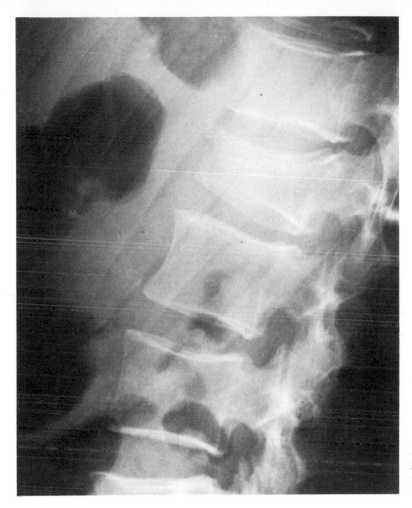

Figure 2-19. Compression fracture of the first lumbar vertebra.

occurs. The bony spinal injury that is potentially unstable or causes spinal cord injury initially presents an entirely different problem in nursing care and management.

THORACIC AND LUMBAR SPINE. A compression fracture of a vertebral body is the most common fracture of the spine (Fig. 2-19). This fracture ordinarily occurs secondary to a flexion injury. The flexion forces cause an anterior wedge compression of the involved vertebral body, with preservation of posterior height and no neurologic damage. In this case, the spine is stable and treatment is basically symptomatic. Complications which may occur as a result of this injury are paralytic ileus and temporary bladder dysfunction secondary to retroperitoneal hemorrhage around the fracture site.

Fractures of the transverse spinous processes (Fig. 2-20) are usually stable but painful, and in general can be treated symptomatically.

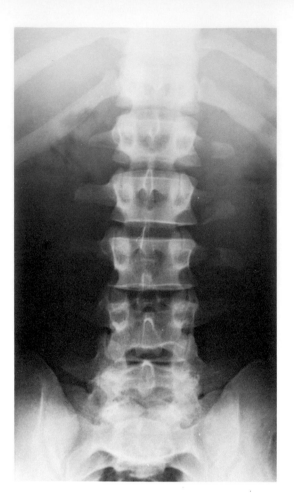

Figure 2-20. Fracture of the first through the third lumbar transverse processes on the left.

The nursing care of patients with these injuries is primarily restoration of normal physiology as soon as pain permits, and prevention of complications. Most patients will receive only an intravenous or clear liquid diet initially. Urine output must be recorded, and catheterization may be necessary. Simple bed exercises that do not reproduce significant pain should be begun as soon as possible, to maintain circulation and muscular function in all involved areas. Gradual mobilization by appropriate instruction in body mechanics and mechanical aids to reduce discomfort should be begun in the early phases. Most of these patients can walk relatively early by using crutches or a walker so that the weight bearing forces are partially transmitted through the upper extremities and shoulder girdle, thereby decreasing the forces passing directly through the thoracic and lumbar vertebrae. The use of some type of external back support (a corset or brace) during ambulation will depend on the physician's preference.

A fracture-dislocation of the spine occurs when tremendous forces are applied to the trunk. This injury is often associated with seat belts. A fracture-dislocation of the spine often causes neurologic damage and may require surgical intervention for reduction or stabilization and decompression.

Traumatic paraplegia is paralysis, both motor and sensory, due to damage to the spinal cord at the level of the skeletal injury. Complications include the development of pressure areas, urinary tract complications and bowel dysfunction.

Early nursing care must consist of prevention of contractures and skin problems by frequent turning and range of motion exercises for all joints, while at the same time careful handling is necessary to prevent further shift in the fractured spine and increasing neurologic damage. Specific nursing actions will of course depend on the level of injury and the medical treatment.

CERVICAL SPINE. Cervical skeletal injuries can occur as a result of flexion, extension, and combinations of flexion, extension, and rotation. If the cord is functionally severed above the level of the fifth cervical vertebra, the injury is often fatal. In addition to the thoracic muscles (chest respiratory muscles) being paralyzed by this injury, the diaphragm, which aids in respiration, is also paralyzed (phrenic nerves of the second, third, and fourth cervical vertebrae). Any cervical skeletal injury carries a potential hazard of serious neurologic damage; therefore, extremely cautious nursing care is essential until the nature and stability of the injury can be adequately assessed. Immobilization must be obtained using sandbags, a cervical collar, or towels. Skeletal traction is applied in the early phases.

The resulting complications as well as the definitive nursing care will depend on the level of injury.

PELVIS. Most pelvic fractures are small undisplaced fractures of the pubic rami (Fig. 2-21) that occur when an elderly patient falls. However, pelvic fractures can range from simple, undisplaced fractures that lend themselves to symptomatic treatment to widely displaced fracture-dislocations of the pelvis secondary to an injury such as a motorcycle or automobile accident. Serious complications such as rupture of the bladder or urethra, injury to the gastrointestinal tract, severance of major vessels with acute blood loss, and sciatic nerve damage may occur as a result of these injuries.

Most undisplaced pelvic fractures are stable and can be treated symptomatically, with an awareness of the possible complications of ileus and bladder dysfunction. The more serious injuries may require skeletal traction for reduction and massive transfusion for severe blood loss: the gastrointestinal and genitourinary injuries may require surgery.

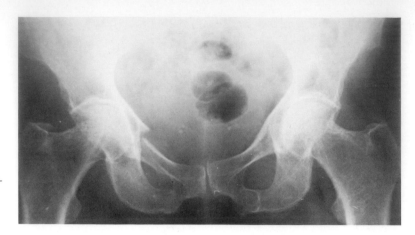

Figure 2-21. Fracture of the pubic ramus on the right.

The nursing care of patients with pelvic fractures is primarily that of restoration of normal physiology as soon as pain permits and the prevention of complications. Simple bed exercises that do not reproduce significant pain should be begun as soon as possible. Most patients with undisplaced pelvic fractures can walk relatively early by using crutches or a walker so that the weight bearing forces are partially transmitted through the upper extremities and shoulder girdle, rather than all passing directly through the pelvis.

Chest Injuries
Open chest wounds require immediate sterile compression dressings to close communication of the thoracic cavity to the outside, and usually immediate surgical treatment is necessary. Closed chest wall injuries require assessment as to whether the mechanics of respiration are significantly disturbed (for example, a flail chest or multiple rib fractures) and whether there are significant internal injuries such as hemothorax, pneumothorax, and pericardial bleeding. These internal injuries must have priority of treatment.

Single rib fractures (Fig. 2-22) are painful, but usually do not cause serious internal injuries and can generally be treated symptomatically with a rib belt and medication for pain. Careful deep breathing several times daily to prevent respiratory infection must be encouraged.

Multiple rib fractures, if extensive enough, can cause a flail chest so that this section of the thoracic cavity has paradoxical motion (collapses in inspiration). This may require skeletal towel-clip traction to a weight for a certain period of time, or a compression-dressing type of immobilization.

Fractures of the sternum can usually be treated symptomatically with observation for respiratory complications unless the fracture is significant enough to interfere with the normal

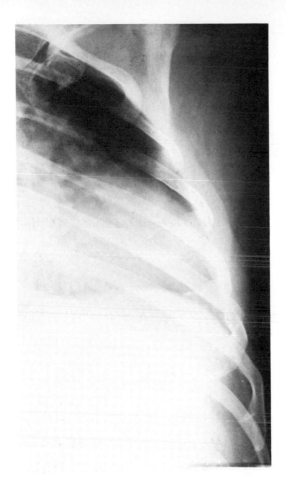

Figure 2-22. Single rib fracture

mechanics of respiration or cause significant pressure on underlying structures.

Upper Limb Injuries

SHOULDER. A fracture of the clavicle (Fig. 2-23) is very commonly seen in children. It is often a greenstick fracture (the tough periosteal sleeve around the clavicle prevents displacement); however, it may be displaced with overriding. Overriding can be accepted, with excellent healing and return of function. This fracture can almost always be treated by simple means involving some type of figure-of-8 splinting to maintain the shoulders in good posture, pain medication for a few days, and gradual, careful activities in a splint for several weeks until the fracture heals. The patient and family need to be told that the physician is aware of the inability to absolutely immobilize a clavicle; when the patient moves about to

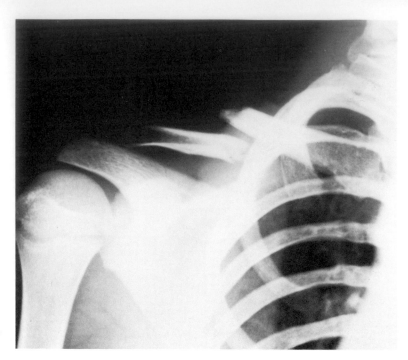

*Figure 2-23. Frac-
tured clavicle.*

change position, he or she may well feel the bones move for
7 to 10 days, until they become "sticky." Similarly, the patient should not be afraid of the immobilization and should
be instructed to insert a finger to push the skin away from
any tight edges of the treatment splint, to pad it if necessary
for comfort, and to let the physician know if the treatment
apparatus is causing intolerable discomfort. Nonunion is rare
and operative intervention is almost never indicated unless
there is a problem in circulation to the overlying skin or damage to the subclavian vessels beneath the fracture site. The patient is treated, not the x-ray.

In a dislocation of the sternoclavicular joint, the clavicle
may dislocate posteriorly behind the sternum or anteriorly
where it joins the sternun. This injury is difficult to diagnose
by x-ray even when clinically suspected. It may require open
reduction, depending on pain, disability, the age of the patient, and other factors.

The acromioclavicular joint (where the clavicle joins the
scapula) is usually injured by a direct fall on the point of the
shoulder. The capsule and ligaments around this joint may be
stretched, sprained, or torn, so that the degree of injury may
range from a sprain to a subluxation or frank dislocation of
the joint. This represents the so-called shoulder separation
(Fig. 2-24). It does not mean that there is any significant injury to the shoulder joint where the humeral head articulates

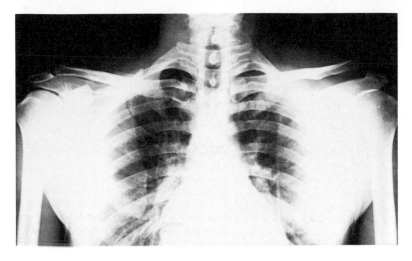

Figure 2-24. Separation of the left acromioclavicular joint.

with the glenoid (scapula). Sprain and subluxation of the acromioclavicular joint can be treated symptomatically with a sling until the ligaments and tissues have healed. Frank dislocations may be treated by open reduction and internal fixation or may be left dislocated in certain cases, depending on the patient's age and occupation and the surgeon's judgment.

Fractures of the scapula are almost always treated symptomatically. Even though the scapula may be severely fractured, it is already encased in a very thick protective muscular splint and good function usually returns with symptomatic treatment.

One of the most common joints to dislocate is the shoulder. Usually the humeral head *dislocates anteriorly* when the arm is in a position of abduction and external rotation: for example, when a person is diving into a pool or putting on a heavy overcoat. In this position the humeral head is forced forward anteriorly and inferiorly, and if the capsular and muscular support is inadequate the shoulder may dislocate. Treatment consists of reduction of the dislocation and immobilization for long enough for the damaged tissues to heal, but mobilization soon enough to prevent permanent limitation of motion and disability. The timing of this treatment naturally varies with the age of the patient. In a relatively old patient the shoulder can be immobilized for much less time than in a young person, since long-term immobilization is more likely to result in permanent stiffness in an older person. Conversely, the shoulder of a younger person can be immobilized for several weeks to allow soft tissues and muscles to heal, with very little danger of any permanent stiffness.

Occasionally a patient will sustain a *posterior dislocation* of

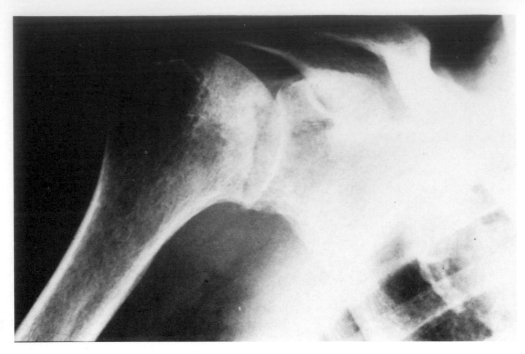

*Figure 2-25. An-
teroposterior
x-ray of posterior
dislocation of the
right shoulder.*

the shoulder (Fig. 2-25). In this case the humeral head slips out behind the posterior edge of the glenoid but at the level of the glenoid. The x-ray is often interpreted as normal. Clinically the arm is locked in a position of internal rotation across the chest. An axillary x-ray view can confirm the diagnosis (Fig. 2-26). Treatment consists of reduction followed by appropriate immobilization.

Inferior dislocation can also occur. The arm may be trapped in an abducted position. Treatment is as already described.

One of the most common fractures in the elderly is a fracture of the surgical neck of the humerus, with relatively slight displacement (Fig. 2-27). These fractures can be treated symptomatically with guided, active assisted range of motion exercises to prevent stiffness, with very little danger of displacement of the fracture or damage from the early motion. After fractures of the neck of the humerus in the elderly, frequently the hemorrhage around the fracture site will work its way to the surface within 24 to 72 hours, resulting in ecchymosis and discoloration around the shoulder, breast, and arm (Fig. 2-28). The patient needs to be informed in advance that this is likely to occur and that it does not indicate a blood clot or any serious complication. The patient and the family

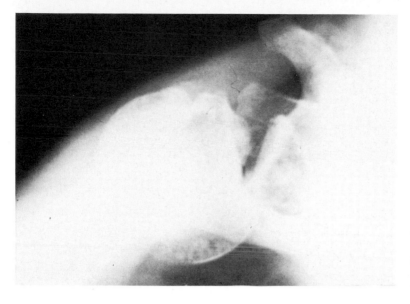

Figure 2-26. Axillary x ray view of posterior dislocation of the right shoulder.

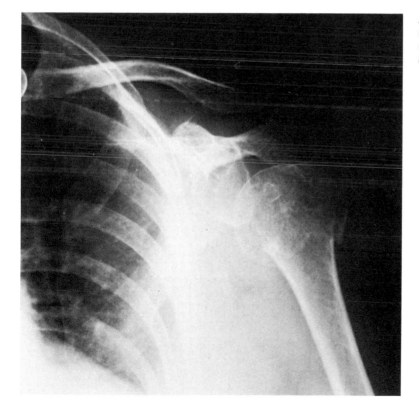

Figure 2-27. Fracture of the surgical neck of the left humerus.

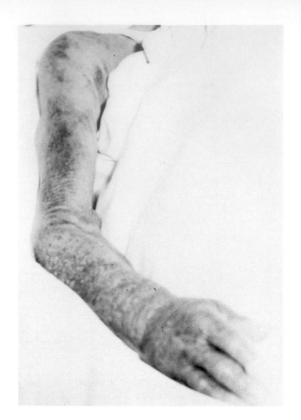

Figure 2-28. Ecchymosis 72 hours after fracture of the surgical neck of the humerus.

should be emotionally prepared to accept this as a natural result of the injury.

The greater tuberosity of the humerus where the rotator cuff inserts may also be slightly displaced and is treated similarly. If it is displaced significantly, operative reduction may be indicated.

Fracture-dislocations of the shoulder (Fig. 2-29) usually require only closed reduction, but occasionally open reduction and internal fixation are necessary (Fig. 2-30).

Rupture of the long head of the biceps (Fig. 2-31) is clinically diagnosed when the patient "makes a muscle": the biceps muscle will bunch up closer to the elbow than on the normal side, because the long head at the upper end has pulled loose. Usually this does not require surgery, depending on the age and occupation of the patient.

Occasionally the rotator cuff muscles are torn. This is a difficult diagnosis to make clinically, but results in limited abduction of the shoulder. This injury requires investigation by an arthrogram, surgery, or both, if initial conservative measures and time do not result in improved function.

HUMERAL SHAFT. Fractures of the humeral shaft (Fig. 2-32)

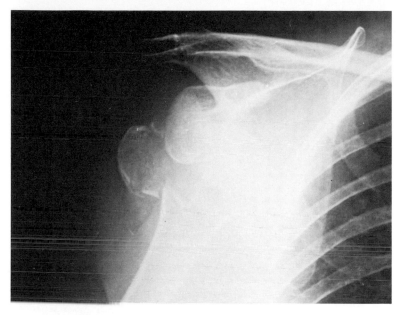

Figure 2-29. Fracture-dislocation of the right shoulder. Note the displaced greater tuberosity.

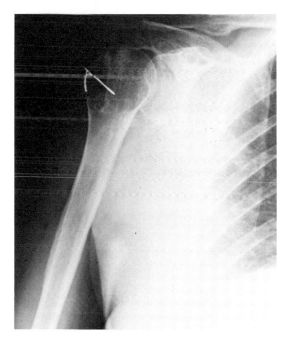

Figure 2-30. The right shoulder after open reduc- and internal fixation of the greater tuberosity.

can usually be managed by gentle reduction under local or general anesthesia to achieve alignment (slight shortening and overriding are entirely acceptable). Alignment is maintained by treatment with a collar and cuff and splinting around the humerus or hanging cast. Nursing care usually requires that the

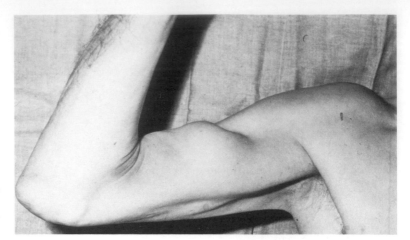

Figure 2-31. Rupture of the long head of the biceps. Note that the muscle bunches up nearer the elbow than is normal.

patient be treated in a sitting or semisitting position so that the upper extremity is essentially suspended by the sling around the neck and wrist, allowing the weight of the arm with the elbow flexed to 90 degrees to maintain acceptable alignment of the fracture. If a nerve injury occurs in fractures of the humeral shaft it usually is the radial nerve that is damaged; therefore, the ability of the patient to extend the wrist and fingers must be assessed.

ELBOW. Supracondylar fractures of the humerus (Fig. 2-33) are very dangerous. These injuries usually occur in children who have fallen, and they are associated with a lot of swelling around the elbow. Treatment usually involves reduction and immobilization in a posterior splint or by means of skeletal (olecranon pin) or skin (Dunlop's) traction. Transfixing Kirschner wires may be used. A supracondylar fracture, regardless of treatment, is very serious and must be watched carefully during treatment for evidence of vascular embarrassment of the forearm. One must be aware at all times of the possibility of development of a volar compartment syndrome with pain, pallor, paresthesias, and pulselessness, indicating ischemia of the forearm muscles secondary to some type of vascular injury due to the supracondylar fracture. Always consider the possibility of the development of Volkmann's ischemic contracture in the forearm after a supracondylar fracture. Clinically it may be difficult to distinguish a posteriorly displaced supracondylar fracture of the elbow from a dislocation of the elbow.

Y-shaped fractures of the lower end of the humerus may lend themselves to internal fixation and early motion, or may require traction treatment. These fractures often result in limitation of motion of the elbow.

Fracture of the lateral condyle and capitellum is one of the

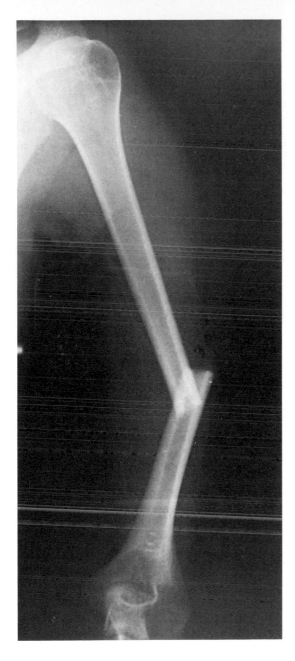

Figure 2-32. Fracture of the shaft of the left humerus.

few fractures in children that may require open reduction. If the ossification center of the injured capitellum does not appear comparable to that of the uninjured elbow, this may represent a fracture through the capitellum with some displacement of the articular surface that cannot be seen on the x-ray. Open reduction may be indicated, since the lateral con-

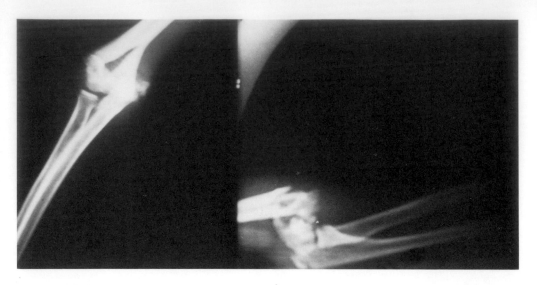

Figure 2-33. Su-
pracondylar frac-
ture of the
humerus.

dylar fragment may rotate up to 90 degrees even though the x-ray may not appear to show great displacement.

In avulsion of the medial epicondyle, good function can result after treatment if the avulsion is not great. Occasionally the epicondyle is avulsed and pulled into the elbow joint, in which case open reduction and internal fixation are indicated.

Dislocations of the elbow are most often posterior, the olecranon being posterior to the humerus (Fig. 2-34). This occurrence is a surgical emergency, since reduction must be accomplished rapidly to prevent edema and serious neurovascular damage. Reduction can usually be accomplished under local anesthesia with gentle manipulation and then temporary immobilization in a posterior splint with the elbow flexed 90 degrees.

Fractures of the olecranon (Fig. 2-35) may require open reduction. If less than half of the olecranon is involved, this may lend itself to removal of the olecranon fragment, repair of the triceps to the remaining portion of the olecranon, and early motion.

Treatment of a fracture of the head of the radius depends on the involvement of the articular surface and the amount of displacement. The orthopedic surgeon decides whether to remove the radial head or leave it in place. Early motion is begun in either case.

The clinical picture of a so-called pulled elbow is usually seen in children under the age of 5 years, when an adult or a sibling has pulled the child by the hand. The child screams, the arm drops to the side, and attempts to actively or passively supinate the forearm cause the child to scream with pain.

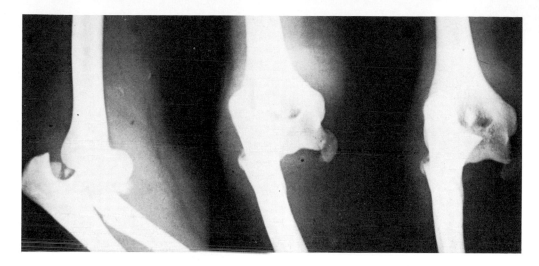

Figure 2-34. Dislocation of the elbow with associated fracture.

Figure 2-35. Fracture of the olecranon.

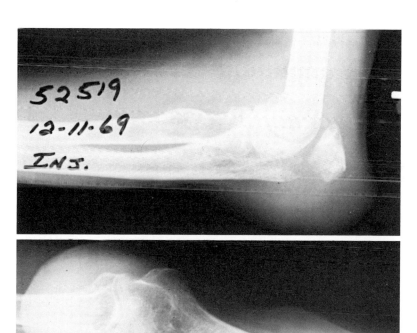

X-rays of the elbow are normal. Reduction is almost always accomplished with gentle traction, flexing the elbow, and exerting pressure over the radial head with marked supination of the forearm as the elbow is flexed. A click can usually be felt, after which the child is able to supinate the forearm. It is thought that in these cases there is some type of synovial or ligamentous structure caught between the radial head and the humerus.

The biceps tendon can also rupture at its insertion in the radius. Clinically this is diagnosed when the patient "makes a muscle"; the biceps will bunch up more proximally than normal when compared with the opposite arm. Flexion will also be somewhat weakened (still present because of the brachialis muscle). Repair of the ruptured biceps tendon is usually indicated, particularly in young persons and manual laborers.

FOREARM AND WRIST. In fractures of the radial and ulnar shafts (Fig. 2-36), displacement often occurs due to the trauma or pull of the forearm muscles. For an excellent functional result in adults, it is very important to have excellent reduction. For this reason, displaced forearm fractures in adults are often treated with open reduction and internal fixation (Fig. 2-37). In children, overriding can be accepted as long as overall alignment is satisfactory; therefore, closed methods are usually satisfactory.

If the ulna is fractured and overriding or angulating and the radius is not, the elbow must be assessed for a dislocation of the radial head at the elbow (a Monteggia fracture) (Fig. 2-38). Similarly, if the radius is fractured and displaced or angu-

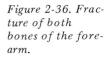

Figure 2-36. Fracture of both bones of the forearm.

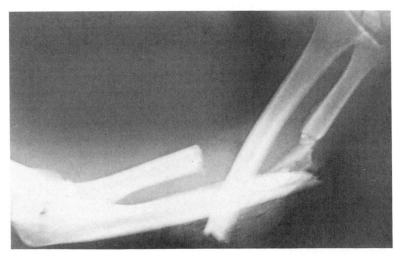

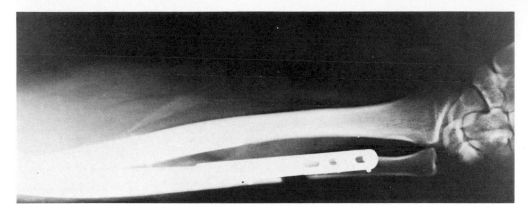

Figure 2-37. Internal fixation of a fracture of the forearm.

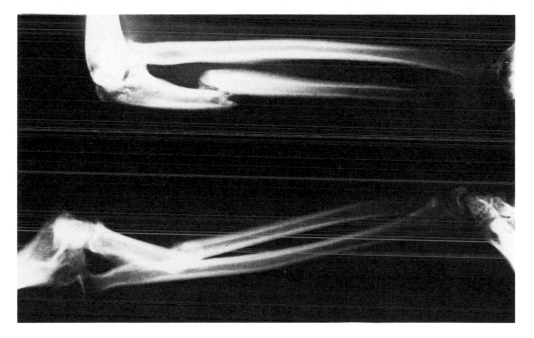

Figure 2-38. Monteggia fracture. Note the dislocated radial head.

lated and the ulna is not, the wrist must be assessed for a dislocation of the radio-ulnar joint.

In adults, by far the most common fracture is a Colles' fracture (Fig. 2-39). This fracture involves the distal radius and often the ulnar styloid process. Usually this fracture occurs with a fall on the outstretched hand. The articular surface of the radius loses its normal volar angulation and is tilted dorsally, with compression of the bone and shortening of the ra-

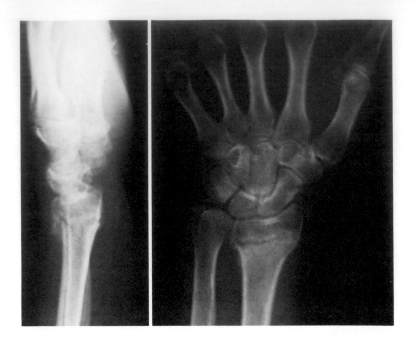

Figure 2-39. Colles' fracture.

dius. A closed reduction is usually satisfactory in the treatment of a Colles' fracture. A reverse Colles' fracture is the so-called Smith fracture, in which the angulation of the articular surface of the radius is volar.

The most common fractures of the forearm seen in children are buckle, torus, and greenstick fractures of the radius and ulna; the bone is crinkled or fractured across but the tough periosteum maintains the bone in good overall alignment. Simple cast immobilization for several weeks to allow healing is adequate.

Displaced fractures of the distal radius and ulna are also common in children. These fractures can usually be treated with closed reduction; if alignment is obtained, even if overlapping is present in the younger child, satisfactory remodeling will occur. Open reduction is almost never indicated.

In an adolescent, the distal radial epiphysis may separate due to injury (Fig. 2-40). This is called a fracture-separation of the epiphysis. Unless displacement is marked, usually immobilization is adequate treatment, since rapid remodeling occurs when a fracture is adjacent to the epiphysis. However, fractures near epiphyses in children may stimulate overgrowth while fractures through or into the epiphyses may damage growth, with subsequent shortening, angular deformity, or both.

CARPAL BONES. Fractures of the carpal bones are rare. The most common and important carpal bone injuries are frac-

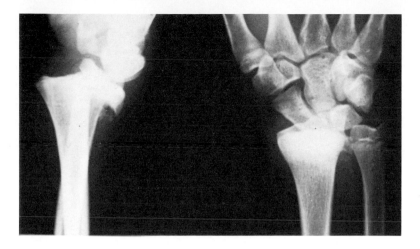

Figure 2-40. Fracture-separation of the distal radial epiphysis.

tures of the scaphoid (navicular) and dislocation of the lunate. After a fall on an outstretched hand a patient may complain of soreness in the wrist. The initial x-rays may be normal. However, if the patient has pain on firm pressure over the anatomic snuffbox on the radial aspect of the wrist (Fig. 2-41), a clinical diagnosis of a possible unseen fracture of the carpal scaphoid (navicular) is made (Fig. 2-42) and the wrist is immobilized. Repeat x-rays are made in 7 to 10 days. At that time, if the scaphoid (navicular) is fractured the fracture line will become evident.

A dislocation of the lunate is a rare injury which is often overlooked on x-rays. If the wrist is painful and swollen and has been injured, one must consider the possibility of a dislocation of the lunate. When this injury occurs, the lunate dislocates on the volar aspect of the wrist; if sought, this can be recognized on x-rays. Median nerve symptoms may be present as the lunate presses against the median nerve in the wrist. Reduction is necessary, and an open procedure may be required.

Dislocations of the radiocarpal joints are rare. More commonly the wrist carpals dislocate around the lunate, which remains in position. This type of dislocation may be associated with a fracture of the scaphoid (navicular) and if so it is called a transscaphoid perilunate fracture-dislocation (the fracture occurs across [trans] the scaphoid and the dislocation occurs around [peri] the lunate). Open reduction may be required.

If the wrist is sprained, clinically it is usually of no real consequence, but one must check for pain over the scaphoid (anatomic snuffbox). If the wrist is painful, one must consid-

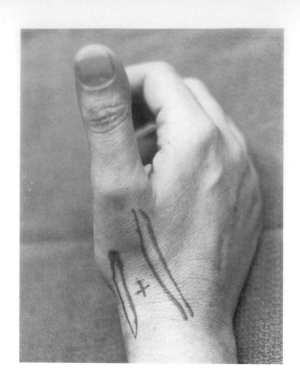

Figure 2-41. Location of the anatomic snuffbox.

Figure 2-42. Fracture of the carpal navicular (scaphoid).

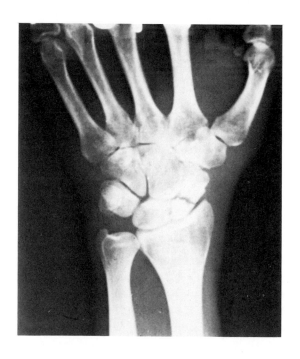

er the possibility of a fracture of the scaphoid (navicular) not seen on the initial x-rays.

HAND. The primary goal in the treatment of hand injuries is return of excellent function, and often this means much more than simply treating the fractures. The results of edema and prolonged immobilization often cause permanent stiffness, contractures, or both, which result in a functionless hand even though the x-rays may show perfect alignment. Therefore, when to start motion in injured fingers and hands to prevent edema and stiffness is decided by the surgeon.

As a general rule, after any type of hand injury a massive compression dressing and splint are used for the first several days after injury or surgery to prevent edema of the hand and fingers. The hand and fingers are immobilized in the so-called position of function, in which the position of the hand is as if a ball were being held. This is done so that if any type of stiffness does occur, the hand will be in the best possible position to allow the return of function.

If articular surfaces are involved in the fingers and small joints of the wrist and hand, frequently open reduction and internal fixation are necessary, since these small joints are often critical in hand function. In addition to assessing injuries to the bones of the hand it is most imperative to assess the neurovascular, muscle, and tendon functions.

Fractures of the bases of the metacarpals are usually not displaced and can be treated by several weeks of immobilization. However, a fracture of the base of the first metacarpal may require open reduction and internal fixation if the saddle-shaped joint is fractured so that there is a fracture-dislocation of the joint.

Fractures of the metacarpal shaft usually are not severely displaced due to surrounding muscle and ligamentous structures, and can usually be immobilized and treated by closed methods. Occasionally, excessive angulation and overriding may necessitate open reduction.

In the so-called boxer's fracture, a fracture of the neck of the metacarpal, the metacarpal head is most frequently displaced slightly into the palm (Fig. 2-43). It can usually be treated with closed manipulation, splinting, and immobilization for 2 to 3 weeks. Even when healing occurs with the knuckle dropped down into the palm, the functional result is often excellent.

In a metacarpophalangeal dislocation closed reduction is generally successful, but occasionally the dislocated metacarpal head, which ordinarily presses into the palm, can be trapped by the capsule and ligamentous structures around the joint; open reduction is then required.

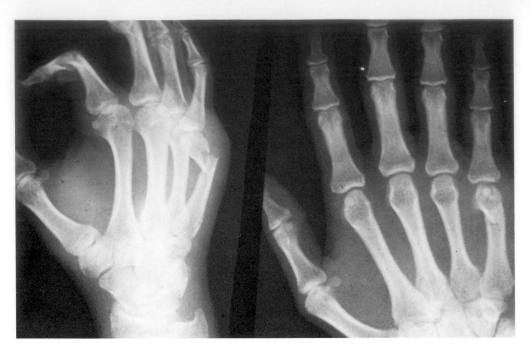

Figure 2-43. Fractured neck of the fifth metacarpal.

Metacarpophalangeal sprains traditionally lend themselves to temporary splinting for 10 to 14 days and then activities are gradually resumed as tolerated.

FINGERS. Phalangeal fractures are usually adequately treated by aligning the finger in the position of function, as if the fingers were holding a ball, with an appropriate splint or a short arm cast. Occasionally internal fixation is required, particularly if a large portion of an articular surface is involved or displaced.

Fractures of the distal phalanx usually occur from an injury such as hitting the phalanx with a hammer. Treatment is for comfort. A painful hematoma may need to be evacuated using a scalpel or a hot paper clip. One should be aware of so-called baseball finger, which is described in the section that follows.

In general, most fractured fingers can be started on motion at approximately 14 to 21 days after injury and are "stuck" by this time regardless of the x-ray appearance.

SOFT TISSUE INJURIES OF THE HAND. The hand is highly vascularized; even though the skin may appear severely damaged initially, it should be cleaned and the wound should be inspected carefully several days after injury, since often more epithelium will survive than one initially expects. When it is obvious that full-thickness skin loss will occur, initial split-thickness skin graft coverage is in order. Skin on the dorsum of the hand and fingers can usually be satisfactorily replaced with split-thickness skin grafts. If skin is lost on the palmar surface of the hand in a patient for whom heavy use and work are necessary, full-thickness flap coverage is usually required.

The neurologic status of the hand must be carefully evaluated in all hand injuries. If a nerve has been severed by a sharp object with little tissue trauma and the wound is clean, a primary repair is usually done. However, in most cases nerve damage occurs when there has been massive tissue damage, and the primary goal is the healing of these tissues, followed by secondary nerve repair.

Flexor tendon injuries in general are more complicated than extensor tendon injuries, particularly if the injury occurs in no man's land, the area between the proximal interphalangeal joint and the distal palmar crease. In this area the tunnel for the flexors is quite small, and suture of tendons in this area often results in scarring and very poor function. Usually injuries in this area are best treated by delayed repair, delayed tendon grafts, or both. Flexor tendon injuries in other areas as well as extensor tendon injuries usually can be treated with primary repair if the wound is a clean, incised one; otherwise, a secondary repair is necessary.

The so-called baseball finger occurs when the extensor to the distal phalanx pulls off, allowing the distal phalanx to flex. This injury necessitates appropriate splinting in extension for several weeks.

Boutonnière deformity refers to the attitude the finger assumes after a rupture of the central extensor slip at the proximal interphalangeal (PIP) joint (Fig. 2-44). The lateral extensor slip drops down, flexing the PIP joint and hyperextending the distal interphalangeal (DIP) joint. This usually requires surgery or some type of special immobilization.

Lower Limb Injuries

HIP. A dislocation of the hip (Fig. 2-45) is most commonly posterior and is usually caused by an automobile accident in which the knee hits the dashboard, forcing the femoral head out of the posterior aspect of the hip joint. When this occurs, the hip internally rotates and is locked in a position of adduction, flexion, and shortening. When a person is seen in the emergency room with the thigh in this position, it almost always is indicative of a posterior fracture or fracture-dislocation of the hip (Fig. 2-46). (Clinically, note an abrasion on the knee.)

An anterior dislocation of the hip is a rare injury. This occurs when the femur is forcefully externally rotated and abducted, causing the femoral head to dislocate through a ruptured anterior capsule of the hip. The lower extremity is

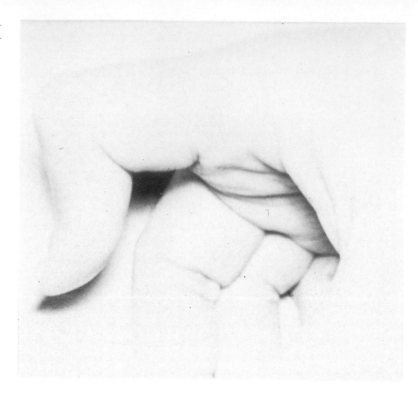

Figure 2-44. Boutonnière deformity of the finger.

Figure 2-45. Dislocation of the left hip.

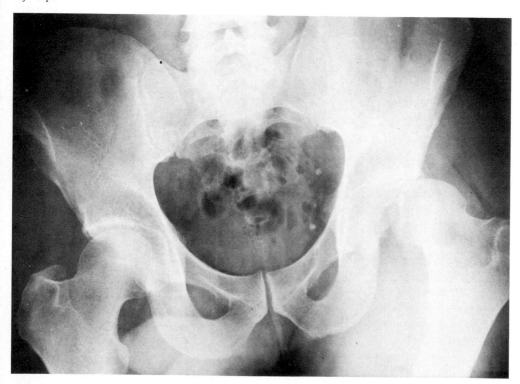

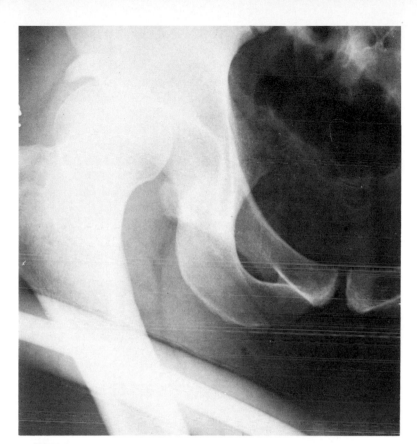

Figure 2-46. Posterior fracture-dislocation of the right hip.

Figure 2-47. Central dislocation of the hip with acetabular fracture.

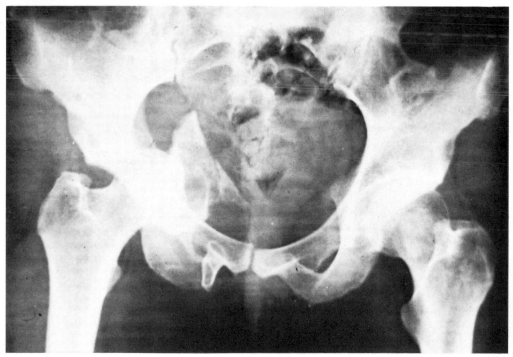

2. Trauma

held in a position of abduction and external rotation and often the femoral head can be palpated beneath the inguinal ligament in the anterior part of the thigh. The femoral artery and nerve which run in this area can be compromised at this point and their function should be assessed immediately.

A central dislocation of the hip also occurs with a central fracture of the acetabulum (Fig. 2-47), the mechanism of injury being a direct blow over the trochanteric area.

The treatment of a dislocation of the hip is immediate reduction, which can usually be accomplished under general anesthesia without open surgery. Occasionally the iliopsoas, the capsule, or both, may prevent reduction, thereby necessitating surgery. Postoperatively, the hip is protected in a stable position until the capsule and soft tissues can heal. Gradual mobilization is then allowed. In central acetabular fractures and dislocations of the hip, because of the instability, skeletal traction for an extended period of time, but with early motion to prevent stiffness, may be the treatment of choice.

Fractures of the neck of the femur are of several different types. A direct fall on the trochanter may produce an impacted fracture of the neck of the femur in good position which allows fairly good function, even in the acute injury phase, and the patient may even walk on the limb. Usually this type of fracture is stabilized without manipulation, with threaded pins to prevent the danger of further displacement. Many fractures of the femoral neck are displaced at the time of injury (Fig. 2-48). If this has occurred, the extremity usually assumes a position of shortening and external rotation due to displacement at the fracture site and muscle spasm which shortens and externally rotates the involved leg. Treatment of displaced femoral neck fractures is either reduction and internal fixation (Fig. 2-49) or removal of the femoral head and replacement by a prosthesis (Fig. 2-50). Which procedure is elected depends on the age of the patient, the type of fracture, and the surgeon's preference and judgment. It is important to remember that the blood supply to the femoral head is obtained primarily from blood vessels around the base of the neck of the femur which run up the femoral neck into the femoral head. Therefore, fractures across the neck of the femur often damage the blood supply to the femoral head enough to cause avascular necrosis of the femoral head at a later date. Just how badly the blood supply is damaged cannot be ascertained at the time of injury.

FEMUR. Intertrochanteric fractures of the femur occur in the area of the femur between the greater trochanter and the lesser trochanter (Fig. 2-51). Here the blood supply is almost

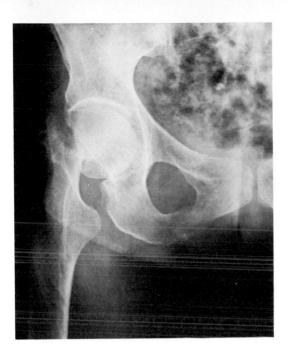

Figure 2-48. Displaced fracture of the right femoral neck.

Figure 2-49. Internal fixation of a fracture of the right femoral neck (Knowles pins).

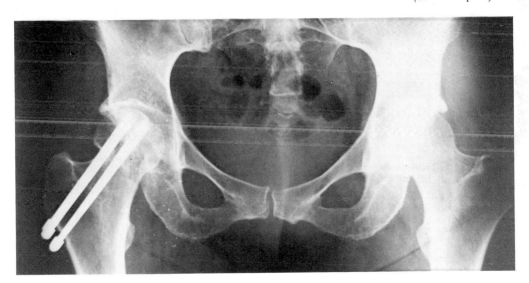

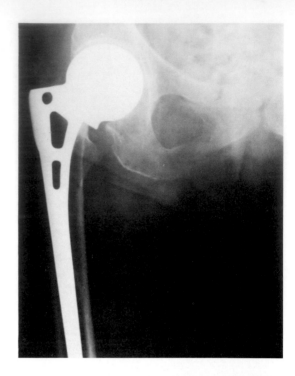

Figure 2-50. Moore hip prosthesis inserted for displaced fracture of the right femoral neck.

Figure 2-51. Intertrochanteric fracture of the left hip.

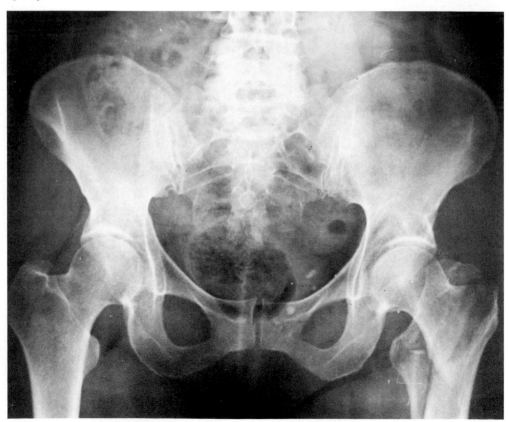

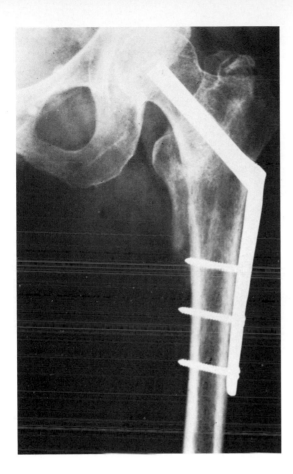

Figure 2-52. Jewett-nail fixation of an intertrochanteric fracture of the left hip.

always satisfactory; therefore, most fractures of this type are treated by open reduction and internal fixation (Figs. 2-52, 2-53), as healing will usually result. Prosthetic replacement is not indicated.

A subtrochanteric fracture of the femur is a fracture just below the trochanteric region (Fig. 2-54). The muscle forces in this area cause problems with maintenance of reduction by closed or open means. Because of this, a special type of fixation device may be used or an intramedullary rod may be inserted as well as a side-plate, with or without a nail. Complications are common because of the concentration of deforming forces tending to displace a fracture in this area into varus.

Isolated avulsion fractures of the lesser trochanter can be treated symptomatically with excellent return of function. Open reduction is not necessary. Fractures of the greater trochanter, which are usually essentially undisplaced, can also be treated symptomatically.

2. Trauma

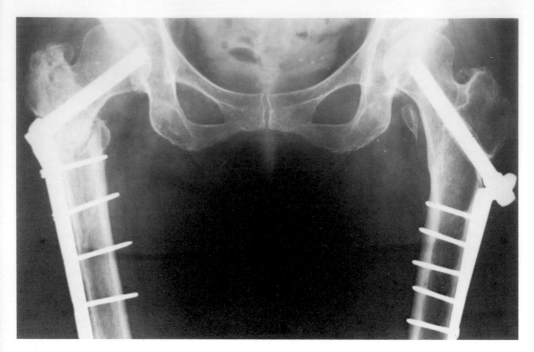

Figure 2-53. In-
tertrochanteric
fractures (left hip
fixed with Mc-
Laughlin type of
nail-plate; right
hip fixed with
Smith-Petersen
nail and Thornton
side-plate.)

Figure 2-54. Sub-
trochanteric frac-
ture of the left
hip.

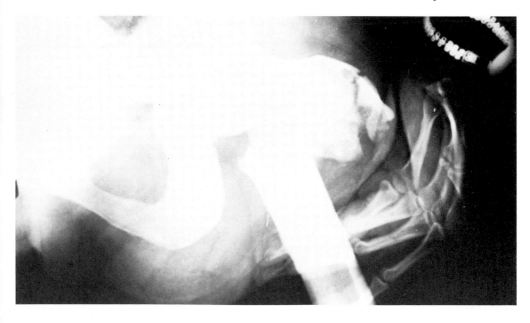

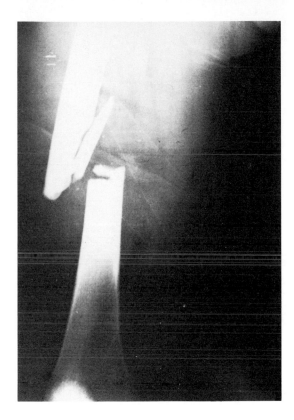

Figure 2-55. Fracture of the shaft of the femur.

Fractures of the shaft of the femur in adults (Fig. 2-55) usually occur from severe trauma such as a motorcycle or automobile accident. One must be alert to shock from pain and blood loss, since one to two units of blood can be lost in the closed femoral fracture. Initial treatment consists of appropriate splinting (usually a Thomas splint, traction, or both) and assessment of blood loss, necessary fluid replacement, and pain. Definitive treatment usually falls into one of the following categories: (1) traction until the fracture is "sticky," progressing to a spica cast or a cast brace; or (2) several days after injury, when the patient's condition is stable, elective open reduction and internal fixation of the fractured femur using an intramedullary rod, side plate, or both. If stable internal fixation can be achieved then early ambulation on crutches is possible.

Fractures of the shaft of the femur in infancy and childhood (Fig. 2-56) are usually treated with traction followed by a spica cast. Overriding of up to 1.5 to 2 cm and a considerable amount of angulation can be accepted with excellent remodeling and return to function (Fig. 2-57). The younger the child, the greater the acceptable deformity; because of this,

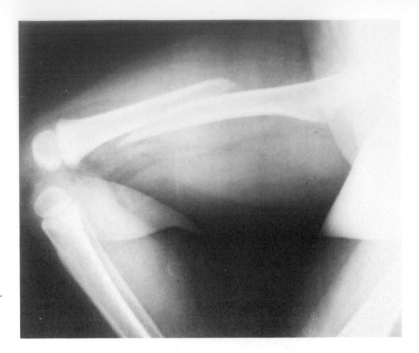

Figure 2-56. Fracture of the shaft of the femur in child.

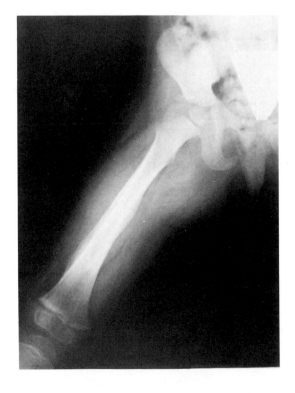

Figure 2-57. Healed fracture of the shaft of the femur in a child. Note remodeling.

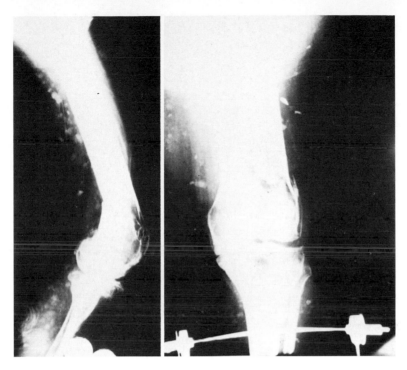

Figure 2-58. Skel etal traction for a supracondylar fracture of the femur.

operative procedures for fractures of the femur in children are almost never indicated.

A supracondylar fracture of the femur is a difficult injury to treat because of the muscular pull on the distal fragment, which not only causes this fragment to rotate but also may impinge on the popliteal vessels and nerves. Alignment is difficult to maintain for the same reason, and usually the knee must be flexed to allow the muscles to relax. Treatment usually involves traction until the fracture begins healing in a good position (Fig. 2-58), or open reduction and internal fixation.

Fractures of the femoral condyles are treated by traction and early motion in traction if alignment can be maintained. Occasionally these injuries may be treated by open reduction and internal fixation, again with motion as early as possible.

KNEE. The extensor apparatus of the knee begins with the quadriceps muscle, which blends into the quadriceps tendon; this tendon inserts into the patella, becoming the patellar tendon and inserting into the tibial tubercle. When this apparatus is shortened, the knee extends. Any injury in the mechanism of the extensor apparatus, such as a rupture of the quadriceps tendon, a displaced fracture of the patella, a

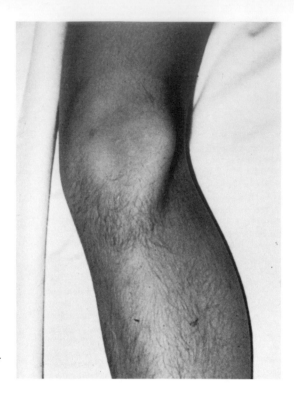

Figure 2-59. Lateral dislocation of the left patella.

rupture of the patellar ligament, or an avulsion of the tibial tubercle, can result in inability to adequately extend and stabilize the knee. This extensor mechanism must be restored to continuity and usually surgical means are required. After repair of the extensor apparatus by whatever methods necessary, the knee usually needs to be protected in extension for at least 3 weeks and then early range of motion exercises can be begun carefully to prevent knee stiffness.

Dislocation of the patella almost always occurs laterally (Fig. 2-59), usually in young girls. Reduction is required, with immobilization to allow the torn retinaculum to heal, followed by quadriceps strengthening exercises. If dislocation recurs, operative procedures may be necessary.

The most powerful supporting ligaments of the knee are the medial and lateral ligaments. These can be ruptured by a severe external force applied to the knee. The medial collateral ligament is ruptured when valgus strain is applied to the knee. In young athletes, when one of these ligaments is completely ruptured open reduction and surgical repair are usually indicated.

The anterior and posterior cruciate ligaments are also supporting structures at the knee. Rupture of these ligaments usually occurs in association with other serious ligamentous and cartilaginous ruptures. Depending on the type of injury, surgical repair, removal of the cruciate ligament, or both, may be indicated. If the ligament is removed, compensation for its removal is achieved by a powerfully developed quadriceps muscle and good development of the hamstrings.

The medial or lateral tibial plateau may be depressed or fractured in association with or separate from a bone injury (Fig. 2-60). Depending on the type of fracture and degree of displacement, treatment usually consists of traction and early motion. Occasionally open reduction and internal fixation may be necessary.

Dislocation of the knee is a rare injury. When it occurs the femur is usually driven posteriorly behind the tibia. All of the ligamentous structures and capsules of the knee are ruptured, and frequently the popliteal vessels are seriously damaged. This injury can result in loss of the extremity. Immediate reduction is indicated, with an investigation of the vascular sup-

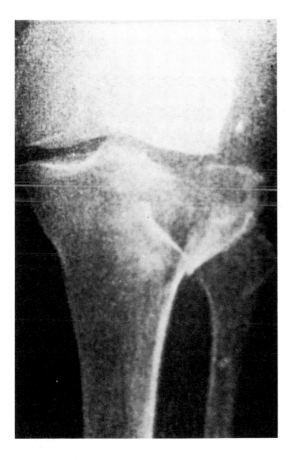

Figure 2-60. Fracture of the lateral tibial plateau of the left knee.

ply to the lower extremity in anticipation of possible surgical repair.

Mild rotatory sprains of the knee can result in effusion and a painful knee. Often one cannot be sure initially whether or not the medial or lateral semilunar cartilages are damaged. The knee must be repeatedly examined during the first week or two after injury and periodically thereafter, to determine if significant injuries to the medial or lateral semilunar cartilages have occurred. Tears in these cartilages usually do not heal and result in a feeling of instability, with recurrent locking and effusion of the knee. If such problems occur, an arthrogram of the knee might be indicated; arthrotomy for removal of the torn cartilage is often necessary.

TIBIA AND FIBULA. Fractures of the tibia and fibula, when due to direct violence, are often associated with more damage to the soft tissues than fractures due to indirect violence (Fig. 2-61). The skin may be opened from without, thereby contaminating the wound. Special attention should be paid to neurovascular function in the foot when the patient is first seen. If the wound is open, a sterile compression dressing should be applied. The leg should always be splinted to avoid further movement and increased soft tissue damage. Wrapping the leg in a large pillow splint is a simple and effective means of splinting while x-rays and further studies are being accomplished. The Thomas splint, often used for a fractured femur, is also satisfactory for temporary splinting of a fractured tibia and fibula. Fractures due to direct violence can cause the tibia and fibula to be fractured at the same level, usually in a transverse or a comminuted manner.

A small amount of energy delivered over a longer period of time can also cause a fracture. The bone can absorb only so much energy before it fractures, and fractures due to indirect violence are usually the result of energy delivered to the bone for a longer period of time, such as a twisting injury while skiing. This type of indirect violence usually produces a closed fracture, the tibia breaking in a spiral fashion and the fibula usually fracturing at a higher level. The skin remains intact. Appropriate splinting as already described is in order.

In a fracture of the tibia only, displacement is usually not as great because the intact fibula gives some stability to the leg. Appropriate evaluation and splinting are in order.

A fracture of the shaft of the fibula usually occurs from direct violence. The interosseous ligament between the tibia and fibula stabilizes the remainder of the fibula, and treatment is usually for pain rather than for the fracture itself. Offset of the fracture is well tolerated and does not have to be corrected. If the patient is not too uncomfortable, an elastic bandage wrapping, elevation, and partial weight bearing

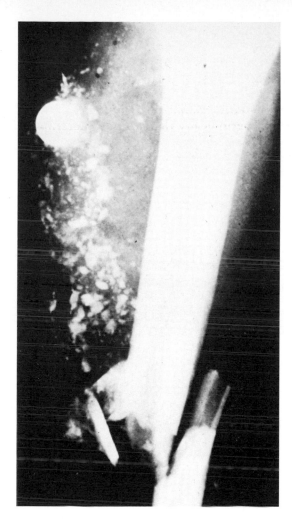

Figure 2-61. Open fracture of the tibia and fibula with soft tissue damage.

with crutches, as tolerated, are in order. However, a cast may be necessary to control discomfort. If the fracture is at the proximal end of the fibula, careful attention should be paid to peroneal nerve function, as this nerve crosses the upper end of the fibula. Similarly, if a cast is applied, care must be taken to prevent pressure in this area from the swelling.

Fractures of the distal end of the fibula are included in the section on ankle injuries.

A fracture of the proximal end of the tibia usually is a result of direct violence. The patellar tendon insertion in the tibial tuberosity often will extend the proximal fragment, causing compromise to the skin overlying the fractured area. The anterior tibial artery penetrates the interosseous membrane in this area and can be damaged at the time of injury or by subsequent swelling. Careful assessment must be made of the integrity of this vessel. Splinting the knee in extension, to relax the pull on the patellar tendon by the quadriceps mechanism, is appropriate.

Children can incur buckle fractures of the tibia and fibula and still limp on the leg. This is especially true in very young children, who cannot tell you where they hurt. In general, fractures of the tibia and fibula in children can be treated with casting. Overriding and slight angulation can be accepted, particularly in the younger child, and excellent remodeling can be expected as growth occurs.

SOFT TISSUE INJURIES OF THE LOWER LEG. A rupture of the Achilles tendon usually occurs in individuals performing activities as usual, such as playing tennis or golf, or walking briskly. This injury occurs most commonly in males. The individual has pain behind the ankle, is unable to forcibly plantar flex the foot, and cannot push up on tiptoe. With a finger, one can often palpate a defect in the Achilles tendon behind the ankle. When the area of the gastrocnemius is squeezed, the foot will plantar flex reflexively if the Achilles tendon is intact. This is known as the squeeze test for Achilles tendon injury. Treatment usually consists of surgical repair of the ruptured tendon, although in certain circumstances this injury may be treated with the foot in a plantar flexed cast for several weeks.

An individual also may be seen with pain in the calf and in the Achilles tendon area who gives a history of feeling as if a golf ball or tennis ball had hit him in the calf. If no defect is palpated in the Achilles tendon and the squeeze test is not positive for an Achilles tear, clinically it is felt that in these cases the plantaris tendon, which runs alongside the Achilles tendon, has ruptured. This is an expendable tendon, and treatment is symptomatic: crutches, elevation, and an elastic bandage wrap.

ANKLE. The most common injury to the ankle is a sprain. This usually occurs when the foot inverts at the ankle joint, the body weight then stretching the ligaments on the lateral side of the foot (the ligaments between the fibula and foot). Swelling and pain occur over the lateral aspect of the ankle. The x-rays are negative except for soft tissue swelling, but one cannot tell from the x-rays whether or not the ligaments have been severely injured; this depends on clinical judgment.

The treatment of a sprained ankle ranges from initial elevation, an elastic bandage wrap, and rapid resumption of full activities to a short leg cast for several weeks to allow torn ligaments to heal. Whether or not a cast is necessary depends on the age and activities of the patient, and the clinical evaluation of the ankle by the treating physician. Occasionally the ligaments are abnormally stretched, and the patient will have frequent, disabling, recurrent inversion sprains of the ankle. These sprains are treated by peroneal strengthening exercises, a lateral heel wedge to prevent inversion of the foot, and occasionally reconstructive ligament surgery.

The talus articulates the foot to the leg. The talotibial joint allows plantar flexion and dorsiflexion of the foot. The talus is contained within the ankle mortise by the distal articular surface of the tibia, the medial malleolus and posterior malleolus, and the articular surface and distal end of the fibula, which comprise the lateral malleolus. Force is applied to the ankle joint through the foot and talus. Whether or not a fracture occurs depends on the strength of the ligaments versus the strength of the bones, and on the mechanism of the injury to the ankle. The most common fracture is an undisplaced fracture of the lateral malleolus of the ankle (Fig. 2-62). This injury is clinically difficult to differentiate from a sprain, since there is tenderness, swelling, and pain over the lateral aspect of the ankle in both injuries. If the medial and lateral malleolus are both fractured, this is described as a bimalleolar fracture (Fig. 2-63). If the medial malleolus, lateral malleolus (fibula), and posterior malleolus (posterior lip of the tibia) are all fractured, this is described as a trimalleolar fracture (Fig. 2-64). The most common ankle fractures are

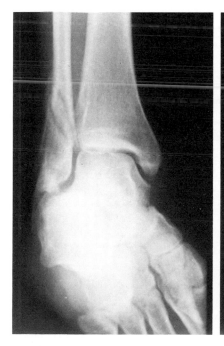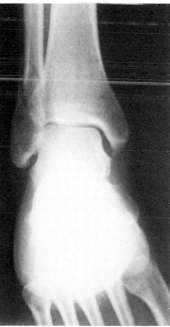

Figure 2-62. Undisplaced fracture of the lateral malleolus of the right ankle.

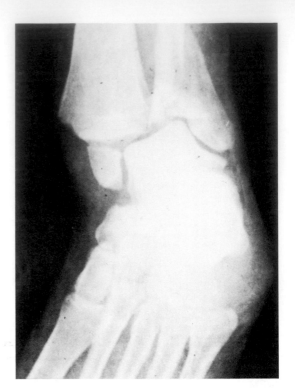

Figure 2-63. Displaced bimalleolar fracture of the left ankle.

produced by external rotation and eversion forces, which break off the lateral malleolus as the talus and foot force it posteriorly and in external rotation. If the force continues, the strong deltoid ligament medially will often pull off and thereby fracture the medial malleolus. With continuing force, the posterior lip of the tibia is fractured also, resulting in a trimalleolar fracture. If the medial malleolus fractures in this fashion, the fracture line is usually transverse. If the medial malleolus is fractured by an inversion injury, the fracture line is usually vertical through the medial malleolus.

Vertical compression injuries can cause a bursting injury to the articular surface of the distal tibia. Often reconstruction of this type of fracture is impossible; the joint is aligned as well as possible, either in a cast or in traction, and early motion is started in the hope of minimizing roughness and arthritic changes in the joint, which may well occur later.

Serious ankle injuries are rare in childhood. Mild sprains do occur, but due to the natural resilience of each structure, severe ligamentous injuries usually do not occur, and ankle fractures are uncommon. The inversion ankle sprain is the most frequent injury. The distal tibial epiphysis can be injured and a fracture-separation at this level can occur. It is usually associated with a fracture of the fibula (lateral malle-

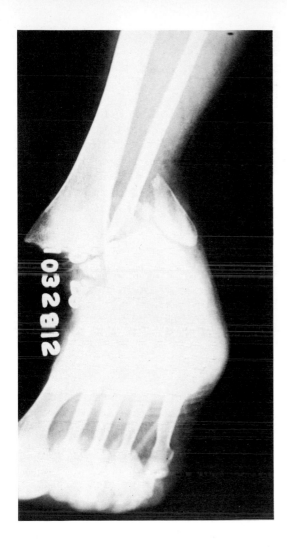

Figure 2-84. Displaced trimalleolar fracture of the left ankle.

olus). The epiphyseal separation can usually be reduced by closed methods. If a fracture occurs through the articular surface of a child's ankle and closed reduction docs not suffice, open reduction and internal fixation may be necessary to restore anatomic relationships. Fractures near epiphyses in children may stimulate overgrowth while fractures through and into the epiphyses may damage growth, with subsequent shortening, angular deformity, or both.

Emergency room treatment of any ankle injury consists of immediate elevation and application of ice to diminish swelling and reduce pain. Anteroposterior, lateral, and oblique x-rays are required to properly evaluate any ankle injury and determine further treatment. Undisplaced lateral malleolar fractures can usually be satisfactorily treated in a short leg walking cast for approximately 6 weeks. Bimalleolar and tri-malleolar fractures are almost always displaced, and because joint surfaces are involved, accurate closed reduction or open reduction and internal fixation are required. Treatment generally then necessitates a long leg cast for 4 to 6 weeks, followed by a short leg cast for an additional 4 to 6 weeks.

FOOT. Fractures of the os calcis (Fig. 2-65) usually occur in individuals who have fallen from a ladder or scaffold. This is a crush type of injury with the fracture involving the subtalar joint. When an injury of this type is seen in the emergency room, one must be particularly aware of the fact that what often happens is that the patient falls, striking the heel and fracturing the os calcis; acutely flexes the back, causing a compression fracture of the spine; and then falls on the hand, causing a Colles' fracture of the wrist. This is a known triad of injuries. Depending on the degree of displacement of the fracture and involvement of the subtalar joint, treatment will range from a massive compression dressing and cast or splinting to reduce swelling, with early motion and prolonged non-weight bearing, to open reduction or percutaneous pin

Figure 2-65. Fracture of the os calcis, lateral view.

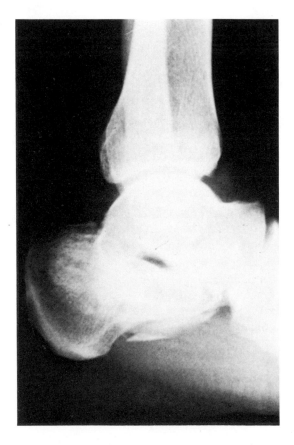

manipulation in an attempt to improve the position of the fractured os calcis. Massive swelling is always a problem with these fractures and initial elevation, compression, and ice are very important in their management. Fractures of the os calcis, regardless of treatment, often cause prolonged disability.

Very high-energy, severe forces are necessary to cause serious injury to the talus. Talar fractures often involve the neck of the talus, resulting in aseptic necrosis of the body of the talus. The main circulation to the body of the talus enters from distal to proximal, and fracture across the neck interferes with the blood supply. Prolonged protection and immobilization are usually required in treatment of a talar fracture.

A midtarsal dislocation requires a severe force, and in order for a dislocation at this level to occur, strong and powerful ligaments have to be ruptured. The initial force may damage the skin and soft tissues considerably. Midtarsal dislocations need to be reduced as soon as possible; often they are unstable and require pin fixation.

Undisplaced fractures of the tarsal bones are rare but can occur. These injuries require immobilization for several weeks. Tarsal fractures, in general, are associated with severe trauma and frequently are open, with severe soft tissue injuries.

Fractures of the metatarsals are usually relatively undisplaced (Fig. 2-66) and can be treated with a walking cast for

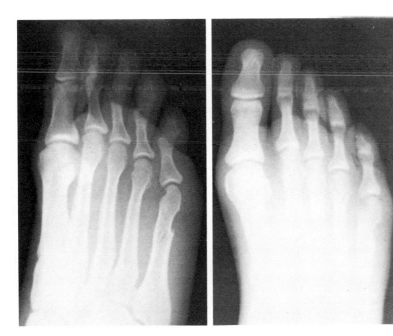

Figure 2-66. Fracture of the shaft of the right fifth metatarsal.

several weeks, or occasionally with a firm-soled shoe after the initial swelling has subsided. If several metatarsals are fractured, a cast is almost always preferable. If marked displacement occurs, reduction and Kirschner wire fixation may be necessary.

TOES. If the phalanges are fractured and the fractures are undisplaced, treatment is symptomatic, with elevation and appropriate protection. If the fracture is angulated, reduction is necessary to allow satisfactory function and shoe wear. Fractures of the great toe often cause more pain than fractures of the smaller toes. Again, the fractures must be properly aligned and this can usually be done by closed methods and local anesthesia. Dislocations of these joints should be reduced as soon as possible and splinted for 2 to 3 weeks.

AMPUTATIONS

Traumatic amputations are generally considered a surgical emergency due to the severed vessels, and amputations for massive trauma are performed as soon as possible to prevent extension of contamination and thus infection.

There is a considerable amount of publicity today about reimplantation of extremities and there is a great deal of medical interest in this possibility. Even in the best of circumstances, limb reimplantation is precarious and the patient is destined to spend months in the hospital and usually to have several surgical procedures. Whether reimplantation should be attempted is a matter of judgment in each individual case; indications for it are exceedingly rare.

SUGGESTED READINGS

Barron, J. N.: Hand injuries and their treatment. *Nurs. Mirror* 136:37–39, April 1973.

Beals, Rodney K., and Hickman, Norman: Industrial injuries of the back and extremities. *J. Bone Joint Surg.* 54 [Am]: 1593-1611, 1972.

Becker, Robert O.: The current status of electrically stimulated bone growth. *Orthop. Nurs. Assoc. J.* 2:35–36, February 1975.

Boericke, Peter H., and Athyn, Bryn: Emergency! *Nursing '75*, pp. 40–47, March 1975.

Bouzarth, William F.: A guide to evaluation of serious head injuries, pp. 21–24. Committee on Trauma, American College of Surgeons, 1974.

Bradley, D.: Fractures of the pelvis. *Nurs. Times* 68:376-379, 1972.

Bradley, D.: Fractures of the ankle joint. *Nurs. Times* 68:1115-1119, 1972.

Bradley, D.: Fractures of the patella. *Nurs. Times* 67:1531-1534, 1971.

Crabbe, W.A.: *Orthopaedics for the Undergraduate*, p. 256. London: Heinemann, 1971.

DePalma, A.F.: *The Management of Fractures and Dislocations* (2nd ed.), p. 901. Philadelphia: Saunders, 1970.

Enneking, W.F.: Management of compound fractures and prevention of infections. *Hosp. Topics* 50:67–68, February 1972.

Esah, M.: Fractures of the tibia and fibula. *Nurs. Times* 68:258-261, 1972.

Harvey, J. Paul: Symposium on the multiply injured patient. *Orthop. Clin. North Am.* 1:10, 1970.

Lea, Robert, and Smith, Lyman: Non-surgical treatment of tendo achillis rupture. *J. Bone Joint Surg.* 54 [Am] : 1398–1407, 1972.

Lindh, Kathleen, and Rickerson, Gail: Spinal cord injury: you can make a difference. *Nursing '74,* pp. 41–45, February 1974.

Marcus, Neal W.: Fractures and dislocations of the spine. *Orthop. Nurs. Assoc. J.* 1:94–95, November 1974.

Miller, Margaret, and Miller, J.H.: *Orthopaedics and Accidents.* London: English Universities Press, 1972.

Pool, Christopher: Colles' fracture: A prospective study of treatment. *J. Bone Joint Surg.* 55[Br] :540–544, 1973.

Rinear, Charles E., and Rinear, Eileen: Emergency bandaging; a wrap-up of better techniques. *Nursing '75,* pp. 29–35, January 1975.

Schultz, R.J.: *The Language of Fractures.* Baltimore: Williams & Wilkins, 1972.

Stone, Kenneth II.: Fractures of the shaft of the humerus. *Nurs. Mirror* 134:26–27, June 1972.

Taylor, A.R., et al.: Traumatic dislocation of the knee. *J. Bone Joint Surg.* 54 [Br] :96–102, 1972.

Wagner, Mary M.: Assessment of patient with multiple injuries. *Am. J. Nurs.* 72:1822–1827, 1972.

Webb, Kenneth J.: Early assessment of orthopedic injuries. *Am. J. Nurs.* 74:1048–1052, 1974.

Wells, Leslie B.: Seven steps to take in orthopedic emergencies. *R.N.* 37: OR/ED 14–18, October 1974.

Whitehead, D.J.: Emergency care in orthopedic injuries. *Nurs. Clin. North Am.* 8:435–440, 1973.

Wray, G.: Injuries of the spinal cord: Primary nursing management. *Nurs. Times* 70:663–666, 1974.

3. COMMON DISEASE PROCESSES AND CONDITIONS

This chapter consists of short summaries of the common disease processes or conditions that affect the normal functions of the neuromusculoskeletal system. There are many excellent textbooks available that explore these processes and conditions in more depth; the reader is directed to those textbooks for additional information.

CONGENITAL DISORDERS

By definition, congenital disorders are present at birth, although they may not be recognized until much later in life. The most commonly seen of these disorders will be discussed; however, the list is not exhaustive.

Congenital Dislocation of the Hip

Congenital dislocation of the hip is one of the most common of the congenital disorders.

Cause. Although the actual cause is not known, there are many factors known to be involved, the hereditary factor being the most distinct. Females are more commonly affected than males.

Pathology. The femoral head may be subluxated or completely dislocated out of the acetabulum; the acetabulum is usually shallow and may be vertical due to the lack of normal pressure by the femoral head.

Clinical Findings. Unfortunately, this abnormality may not be noticed until the child begins to walk. This omission can be avoided if nurses, as well as other members of the health team, routinely examine all babies in the newborn nurseries and in other such clinical situations for this abnormality.

The assessment of this condition should take into account all of the following: When a child is lying on his back, the thigh folds seen are normally symmetrical; however, in a subluxation or dislocation, the folds are asymmetrical or there may be an extra one on the affected side (Fig. 3-1). With the child prone, the buttock fold on the affected side is usually higher (Fig. 3-2). In a subluxation or dislocation, abduction of the affected hip is restricted. This is the most

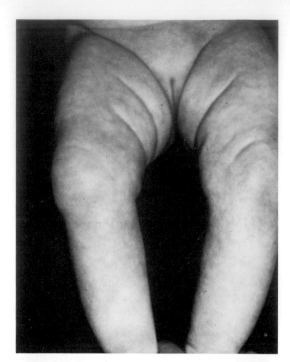

Figure 3-1. Asymmetric thigh folds. Note extra fold on right.

Figure 3-2. Note asymmetric folds; one buttock fold is higher than the other.

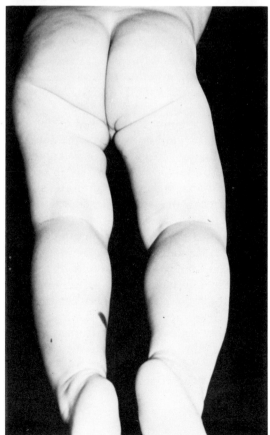

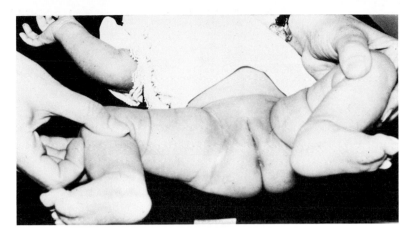

Figure 3-3. Note limited abduction of the left hip.

easily demonstrated finding. Flex the hips 90 degrees and let the legs drop toward the table. If one side is limited (Fig. 3-3) this may be a sign of a dysplastic or dislocated hip. The most frequently used diagnostic test for congenital dislocation of the hip in the newborn is the test for Ortolani's sign. The examiner places the child in the supine position and then grasps the upper part of each thigh with the fingers on the anterolateral aspect and the thumb anteromedially; the child's knees are fully flexed and the hips are flexed to a right angle. Each thigh is steadily abducted toward the table while forward pressure is applied behind the greater trochanter with the middle finger, a palpable or audible click may occur as a dislocated hip is reduced. A positive Allis sign in a unilateral dislocation is demonstrated with the infant on his or her back, with the knees flexed and the feet resting on the table; the knee on the affected side will be lower. There is either real or apparent shortening of the affected side. In a complete dislocation there will also be telescoping of the affected limb; the limb can be displaced by pushing and pulling, and the femoral head palpated as this occurs. In all cases the findings are more prominent in a complete dislocation.

If the congenital dislocation is not diagnosed in early life and the child begins walking, the gait for both unilateral and bilateral dislocation is distinctive. In a unilateral dislocation the child compensates by swaying the body toward the affected side so that the center of gravity is thrust over the femur. In a bilateral dislocation, the swaying from side to side produces a duck-waddle gait. A bilateral dislocation is usually diagnosed later than a unilateral one, since at walking age, the gait is symmetrical in bilateral dislocation and may be considered normal.

X-ray Studies. X-rays are generally made with the hip in several positions, including neutral, maximum abduction, and frog-leg. The x-ray findings in these conditions vary depending on the severity; however, the characteristic findings include displacement of the femoral head, widening of the acetabulofemoral space, a shallow acetabulum with its roof almost vertical, and delayed ossification of the femoral head. Because the femoral head is cartilaginous and its position in relationship to the acetabulum is difficult to determine from standard x-rays, an arthrogram may be performed. The arthrogram will give more information concerning the position of the femoral head, the depth of the acetabulum, and the position of the capsule.

Treatment. The treatment varies with the age of the child and the severity of the problem. During the first year, if only subluxation is found it is treated by placing the hips in abduction and seating the femoral head in the acetabulum by some external device. This treatment usually achieves normal development of the acetabulum by the normal pressure of the femoral head. A dislocated hip must first be reduced and this position held for a longer period of time, usually in a plaster cast. Although closed reduction and casting after the age of 1 year may still be attempted, the results are usually less satisfactory. It should be noted that in some cases skin or skeletal traction may be necessary to relax the soft tissue structures surrounding the hip before closed reduction is attempted. A surgical procedure may be necessary to correct the deformity and is usually done in cases detected after the age of 3 years, or earlier if indicated. The choice of procedure will of course depend on the existing condition.

Congenital Coxa Vara

Congenital coxa vara is any condition in which the neck-shaft angle of the femur is less than the normal of about 125 degrees (Figs. 3-4, 3-5).

Cause. Although this condition may be due to a congenital lack of ossification of a portion of the femoral neck, which causes a gradual bending of the femoral neck, there are other acquired conditions which also result in coxa vara.

Clinical Findings. In this condition there is true shortening of the limb. Coupled with a deficiency of the hip abductors, this leads to a limp. Findings are identical with those seen in congenital dislocation of the hip except that in coxa vara there is no piston mobility, as the head is held firmly in the socket.

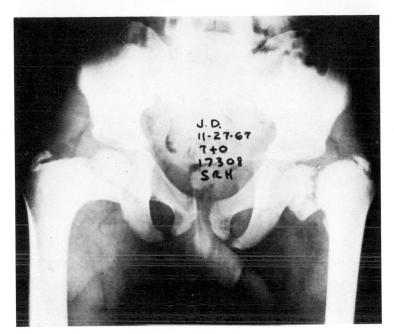

Figure 3-4. Coxa vara of the left hip.

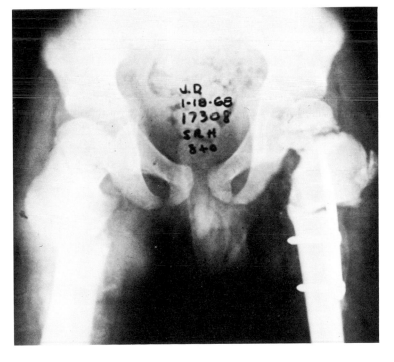

Figure 3-5. Coxa vara corrected by osteotomy.

Osteogenesis Imperfecta

Osteogenesis imperfecta is a congenital affection in which the bones are abnormally soft and brittle (Fig. 3-6).

Cause. This is a hereditary, developmental condition. The onset may occur at any time from before birth to late adolescence. It rarely occurs in adults.

Pathology. Although the primary defect is the failure of formation of osteoblasts, formation of bone by the periosteum is also deficient. The bones are shorter and thinner than normal. Trabeculae are sparse and the cortex of the bone is very thin. There is abnormality of the medullary canals. The deformities seen are a result of fractures and bending.

Clinical Findings. This condition may range from mild to severe. The number of fractures varies, and fractures may be spontaneous. Although healing occurs, it is usually with deformity. With advancing age there is a decreased tendency to fracture. Other characteristics of this condition are dwarfing

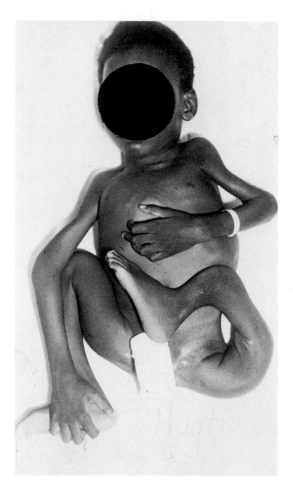

Figure 3-6. A child with severe osteogenesis imperfecta.

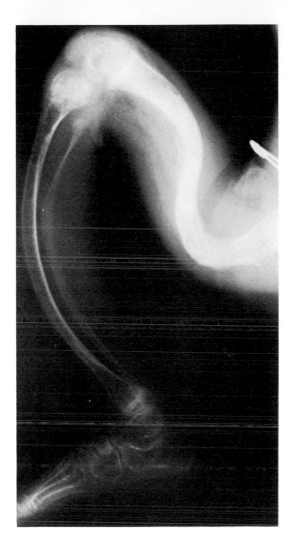

Figure 3-7. X-ray of the right lower extremity in a patient with osteogenesis imperfecta.

caused by the deformities, deafness, laxity of joints, feeble muscles, a broad skull, and poorly calcified teeth.

X-ray Findings. The skeleton is osteoporotic in appearance and the long bones appear thin and elongated (Fig. 3-7).

Treatment. The child must be protected from fractures. Severe deformities may be corrected surgically by osteotomies with intramedullary fixation.

Hereditary Multiple Exostoses

Hereditary multiple exostoses is a condition in which there is formation of many osteocartilaginous exostoses at the metaphyses of long bones. The cause is unknown, although there are many theories as to etiology.

Pathology. The exostoses develop at the growing ends of long bones, first occurring near the epiphyseal cartilage and being displaced along the shaft with growth. When skeletal growth stops there is no more growth of the exostoses.

Clinical Findings. These irregular, hard prominences may be visible or only palpable. They also may be tender. Muscle weakness, paresthesia, or numbness may occur due to pressure on nerves. If an asymptomatic exostosis suddenly becomes enlarged and painful, malignant degeneration must be suspected.

X-ray Findings. The bones are broad and poorly modeled in severe cases. Bony outgrowths are seen that point away from the bone and are conical, spiked, or globular in shape.

Treatment. Excision of an exostosis becomes necessary if it is constantly subjected to injury, causes deformity, or creates pressure on other structures, or if malignancy is suspected.

Achondroplasia

Achondroplasia is a condition in which there is marked shortening of the limbs and thus dwarfing (Figs. 3-8, 3-9).

Cause. The cause is unknown, although there is a hereditary tendency. Females are more commonly affected than males.

Pathology. The long bones are chiefly affected. The process of ossification at the epiphyseal growth plates is disturbed, but periosteal ossification proceeds normally. The base of the skull is fused and short, but the rest of the skull develops normally.

Clinical Findings. The condition is usually apparent at birth or shortly thereafter. The limbs are strikingly short and out of proportion to the trunk. There is a typical trident appearance of the hand. There is no mental impairment, and sexual development is normal.

Vitamin D-Resistant Rickets and Renal Tubular Rickets

Vitamin D-resistant rickets and renal tubular rickets result in defective calcification of growing bone (Fig. 3-10).

Cause. Both disorders are hereditary.

Pathology. In vitamin D-resistant rickets the primary defect is not clearly understood. However, it is felt to be a failure either of normal reabsorption of phosphate by the renal tubules or of the absorption of calcium from the intestine. In renal tubular rickets the primary defects are a failure of the proximal renal tubules to reabsorb phosphate, glucose, and certain amino acids in the normal way, and an excessive loss of phosphate in the urine that leads to the depletion of the bone phosphate.

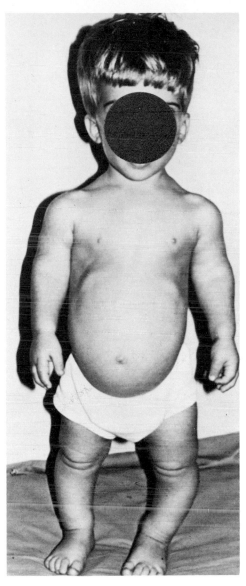

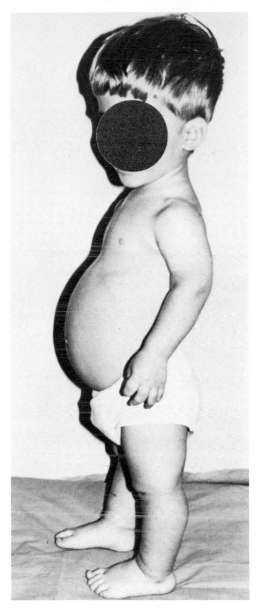

Figure 3-8. Anteroposterior photograph of an achondroplastic child.

Figure 3-9. Lateral photograph of an achondroplastic child.

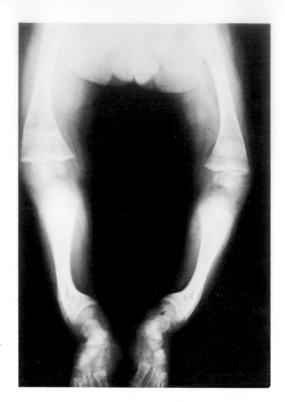

Figure 3-10. Deformities from vitamin D-resistant rickets.

Clinical Findings. The general health of the child is impaired. A large head, retarded skeletal growth, curvature of long bones, deformity of the chest, and enlargement of the epiphyses are present.

X-ray Findings. The vertical depth of the epiphyseal lines is increased and the epiphyses are widened laterally. The ends of the shaft are cupped and an abnormal curvature of the bones may be noted.

Treatment. In vitamin D-resistant rickets, administration of massive doses of vitamin D corrects the adverse bone changes. In renal tubular rickets, the intake of calcium, phosphate, and vitamin D should be increased.

Arthrogryposis Multiplex Congenita

Arthrogryposis multiplex congenita is characterized by stiff, deformed joints of the extremities caused by defective development of muscles.

Cause. The etiology of this condition is unknown, although there is a marked hereditary tendency.

Pathology. The muscles of the extremities are aplastic, with fibrofatty tissue replacing the muscle fibers in many cases. The anterior horn cells may be reduced in number and size in the central nervous system, and the brain may be underdeveloped.

Clinical Findings. The spine is usually not involved, but the condition may be exhibited in one or all four of the extremities. In the upper extremity, fixed deformities may occur in any position; however, most commonly the wrists and fingers are flexed, the forearms are pronated, the elbows are extended, and the arms are internally rotated. Deformities of the lower extremity usually include flexion and internal rotation of the hips, flexion or extension of the knees, and pronounced equinovarus deformity of the feet. The joints appear large in contrast to the small affected limb. There may be subluxation or dislocation of the joints.

Treatment. Correction of the deformity may be attempted by manipulation and serial application of casts; however, recurrence of the deformity is usual. Rehabilitation is less than satisfactory.

Neurofibromatosis

Neurofibromatosis is characterized by pigmented areas on the skin (café-au-lait spots) and multiple neurofibromas along the

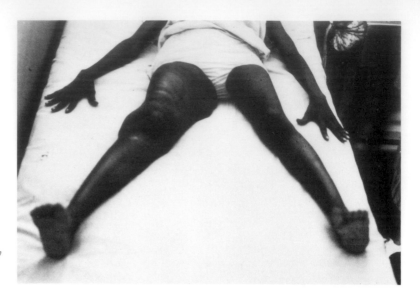

cranial or peripheral nerves. There may also be enlargement of a limb and skeletal changes (Fig. 3-11).

Cause. This is a hereditary condition that may appear at birth or at any time later in life.

Pathology. The neurofibromatous nodules consist of connective tissue arranged in whorls, with a few nerve fibers. They usually are not adherent to surrounding structures.

Clinical Findings. This condition may be manifested in a variety of ways. Skin lesions may be pigmented spots, either flat or raised. Multiple neurofibromas may occur wherever there is a peripheral nerve, and they may be subcutaneous, subperiosteal, endosteal, or intraspinal. Pain and disturbance of function depend on the site. Skeletal changes may result from external pressure or erosion as well as from direct involvement of bone, and irritation or damage to epiphyseal longitudinal growth (Fig. 3-12). Scoliosis is a common occurrence in this condition. Enlargement of part or all of an extremity (elephantiasis) may also occur.

Treatment. Surgical excision of the tissue is performed. Surgical correction of the scoliosis is usually necessary.

Klippel-Feil Syndrome

Klippel-Feil syndrome is a congenital deformity of the cervical vertebrae. The etiology is unknown.

Pathology. There is shortening of the cervical spine due to the reduced number of vertebrae and the fusion of several spinal segments. There are no articulating processes and the intervertebral foramina are narrowed and may encroach on

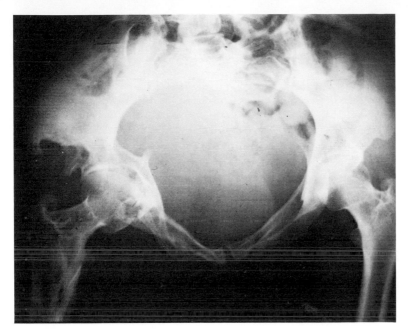

Figure 3-12 Skeletal changes in the right pelvis and hip in a patient with neurofibromatosis.

the nerve roots. This deformity of the cervical vertebrae may result in torticollis, kyphosis, or scoliosis which will cause other symptoms. Spina bifida is frequent.

Clinical Findings. Usually the patient has a short neck and low hairline. Neck motion is limited. The neurologic signs and symptoms vary.

X-ray Findings. These range from the fusion of two or more vertebrae to severe malformations.

Treatment. Some cases are asymptomatic and do not require treatment. Mild nerve root irritation of short duration may be treated with traction or a collar. Neurologic signs and symptoms may require decompression of the nerve root. Surgical correction of the deformity may be necessary depending on its severity.

Congenital High Scapula (Sprengel's Deformity)

Congenital high scapula, or Sprengel's deformity, is a permanent elevation of the shoulder girdle. The etiology is unknown.

Pathology. During embryonic life, there is a failure of the scapula to descend to its normal thoracic position.

Clinical Findings. The scapula is abnormally high. Shoulder abduction is limited because the scapula does not rotate freely.

Treatment. In some cases no treatment is necessary; however, other cases may be treated operatively.

Cervical Rib

Cervical rib is a congenital overdevelopment of the costal process of the seventh cervical vertebra. The cause is unknown.

Pathology. There may be a small bony protrusion or a complete supernumerary rib, unilateral or bilateral.

Clinical Findings. A cervical rib may not cause symptoms, but if they do occur it is usually during early adult life. Neurologic manifestations of the condition include pain and paresthesias in the ulnar side of the forearm and hand; motor weakness of the hand, with decreased ability to carry out finer movements; and sometimes an area of sensory impairment. The vascular manifestations include coldness, pallor, cyanosis, and a weak or absent radial pulse.

X-ray Findings. A cervical rib is seen extending from the seventh cervical transverse process.

Treatment. Surgical removal of the rib may be necessary if symptoms are severe. However, in many cases conservative treatment using an exercise program to increase the tone of the muscles of the arm suffices.

Talipes Equinovarus

Talipes equinovarus describes a congenital clubfoot. The foot is in a position of plantar flexion and inversion (Figs. 3-13, 3-14). The less common types of foot deformities are calcaneovalgus (the foot is in a position of eversion and dorsiflexion); calcaneovarus (the forefoot is dorsiflexed and the heel and forefoot are inverted); and equinovalgus (the foot is in a position of plantar flexion and eversion). Although there are many theories, the etiology is unknown.

Pathology. In talipes equinovarus there is underdevelopment of the muscles of the affected leg as well as abnormal development and displacement of the soft tissues of the foot. The navicular and os calcis are displaced. In the beginning the bony structures are normal; however, as they adapt to the abnormal position they become deformed. In the remaining types of foot deformity, a definite pathological process cannot be ascertained.

Clinical Findings. The deformity is as previously described. A tight heel cord and tight plantar structures are present. Obviously deficient musculature of the leg is seen as well as internal tibial torsion.

X-ray Findings. In talipes equinovarus the scaphoid, cuneiform, metatarsals, and os calcis are displaced medially with respect to the talus. The entire foot is in equinus. In cases of calcaneovalgus deformity the x-rays document the dorsiflexed and valgus position of the foot.

Treatment. Conservative treatment consists of manipulation

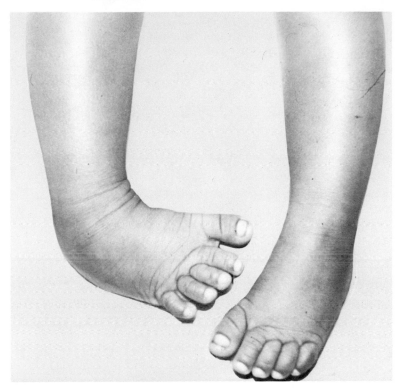

Figure 3-13. Right clubfoot.

Figure 3-14. Bilateral untreated severe clubfoot.

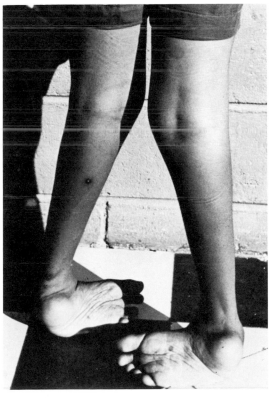

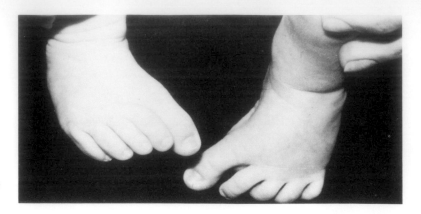

Figure 3-15. Bi-lateral metatarsus varus.

and casting followed by special shoes or devices. Soft tissue or bone surgery may be necessary to correct the deformities.

Metatarsus Varus

Metatarsus varus consists of adduction and inversion of the forefoot, the heel being normal (Fig. 3-15).

Pathology. The great toe and the first metatarsal are pulled medially by the abductor hallucis muscle. The anterior tibial muscle pulls the fore part of the foot into inversion.

Clinical Findings. The foot may appear normal at birth, with the deformity becoming apparent in later weeks. An adduction deformity of the forefoot is seen. The condition must be recognized before the deformity is severe and fixed.

X-ray Findings. The great toe may be widely separated from the second toe. The metatarsals are adducted.

Treatment. Conservative treatment consists of manipulation and casting followed by special shoes or devices. Soft tissue or bone surgery may be necessary to correct the deformity.

Congenital Deformities of the Spine

Congenital deformities of the spine can vary from absence of certain portions of the spine, as in congenital absence of the sacrum with associated severe neurologic deficit, to minor alterations in structure, such as a spina bifida occulta having no clinical significance whatsoever.

Pathology. Failure of fusion of the posterior bony vertebral structures may be associated with underlying neurologic abnormalities and herniation of neural tissues and their coverings through the posterior spinal defect. If the meninges protrude through the posterior spinal defect but no neural tissue is included, then this is called a *meningocele*. If neural elements are also included in the posterior herniation, then it is a *myelomeningocele*. There is often a distal neurologic deficit when a myelomeningocele is present. Congenital fusion of vertebrae can occur, causing shortening of the spinal segment: for example, the congenitally short neck or Klippel-Feil syndrome (congenital synostosis of the cervical vertebrae). Vertebral bodies can be congenitally maldeveloped: for example, hemivertebrae or congenital fusion of several of the vertebrae along one side, resulting in a lateral curvature of the spine or congenital scoliosis. Certain congenital abnormalities of the spine may only be detected later in life, when they are manifested by neurologic problems in the lower extremity secondary to damage to the intraspinal neural structures as growth occurs. For example, diastematomyelia is characterized by an osseous or fibrocartilaginous septum transversing the spinal canal and dividing a part of the cord or cauda equina. As the individual grows the spinal cord cannot normally ascend and traction is exerted on it. The gradual increase in traction on the cord may cause progressive neurologic problems in the lower extremities. Myelography is necessary to diagnose this particular condition.

Treatment. Treatment varies with the condition; it may be conservative or surgical.

Other Congenital Disorders
See Table 3-1 for the clinical characteristics of other common congenital disorders.

INFLAMMATORY DISEASES
Rheumatoid Arthritis
Rheumatoid arthritis is a chronic systemic disease characterized by inflammatory changes in the soft tissue surrounding the joint and often severe joint involvement.

Cause. Many theories have been advanced, including metabolic, endocrine, infectious, and allergic causes of this disease; however, the etiology is unknown.

Pathology. The synovial linings of joints and articular structures become inflamed and swollen with increased synovial fluid. Granulation tissue spreads from the inflamed tissues into the joint, destroying the bone and cartilage. During the acute inflammatory stages, the ligamentous structures become lax, and reflex muscle spasm may produce contractures.

Clinical Findings. Slight swelling and tenderness of a few joints is first noticed. Then there is gradual development of symmetrical involvement. The proximal finger joints are more commonly involved than the distal joints. Joint pain, instabil-

Table 3-1

Congenital Deformity	Clinical Characteristics
Cleidocranial dysostosis	Mild degree of hydrocephalus may be present; small maxilla, large mandible; clavicle may have defect or be devoid of bone; slender build with large head; widespread spina bifida occulta is common; deficient ossification of pubic bones
Congenital anomalies of the hand	Syndactylism — webbing of two or more digits Symphalangism — fusion of interphalangeal joints Polydactylism — more than five digits Brachydactylism — decreased length or number of phalanges or shortened metacarpals Lobster-claw hand — three types, all consist of defect in central portion of the hand (Fig. 3-16)
Congenital hallux varus	Medial angulation of the large toe at the metatarsophalangeal joint; first metatarsal bone may be short and thick; accessory bone and toes often associated; varus deformity of one or more of the other metatarsal bones; a firm fibrous band running from the great toe to the base of the first metatarsal may be present
Congenital pseudarthrosis of the tibia	Anterior bowing of the tibia and shortening (Fig. 3-17)
Congenital absence (most commonly seen)	Radius — may be completely or partially absent Fibula — anterior bowing of the tibia Tibia — part or all may be absent
Congenital torsion in lower extremity	Tibial torsion — internal, with the foot placed pointing forward, the patella and knee are rolled outward
Multipartite patella	Present when ossification centers of the patella fail to fuse; may be bipartite, tripartite, or multipartite; usually asymptomatic
Torticollis	Tilting of the head to one side with rotation toward the opposite side; asymmetric shape of face and head
Congenital constricting bands	Often associated with other clinical deformities; transverse indentions of the skin and underlying soft tissues which are well defined and completely encircle extremity at one or more levels
Hyperlaxity of joints	Hypermobility of joints; ability to hyperextend finger joints

ity, contractures, and destructive arthritic changes occur, with crippling particularly in the hands, wrists, knees, elbows, and feet (Fig. 3-18); however, all joints of the body may be involved. Systemically the patient may have anemia with gradually increasing weakness, general debility, and an eleva-

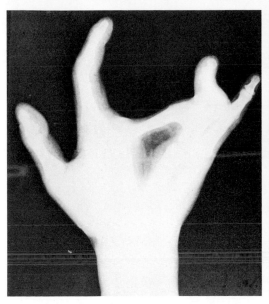 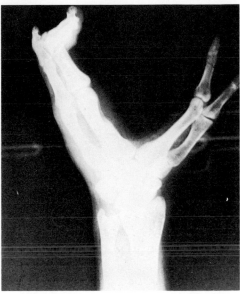

Figure 3-16. Congenital lobster-claw deformity of the hand.

Figure 3-17. Congenital pseudarthrosis of the tibia.

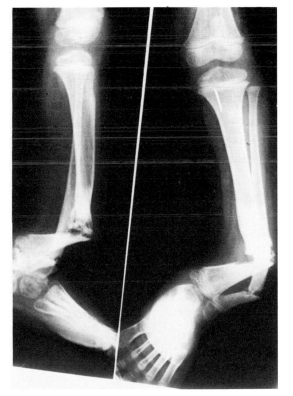

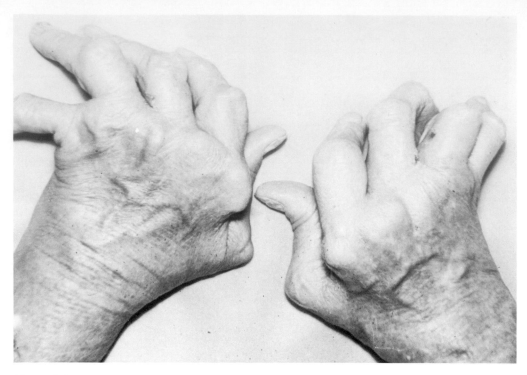

Figure 3-18.
Hands of a patient
with rheumatoid
arthritis.

ted temperature. Subcutaneous inflammatory nodules may develop, usually near the elbow.

Treatment. Treatment consists of an optimal diet, appropriate splinting to prevent joint deformities, rest balanced with exercises, and drug therapy including antiinflammatory drugs, gold salts, corticosteroids, immunosuppressive drugs, and intra-articular corticosteroid injections (these do not cause the deleterious effects of long-term systemic corticosteroids). Surgical intervention may be necessary to arrest the deformity or to correct existing deformity by means of an arthroplasty. Often multiple surgical procedures are required.

Marie-Strümpell Arthritis

Marie-Strümpell arthritis is a progressive inflammatory disease of the spine and larger joints that leads to ankylosis and deformity (Fig. 3-19).

Cause. The cause is unknown, although many theories have been advanced with respect to endocrine, metabolic, infectious, and mechanical factors. This disease occurs primarily in males.

Pathology. Fibrous and bony bridging, especially between the vertebral segments, is frequent, producing a so-called bam-

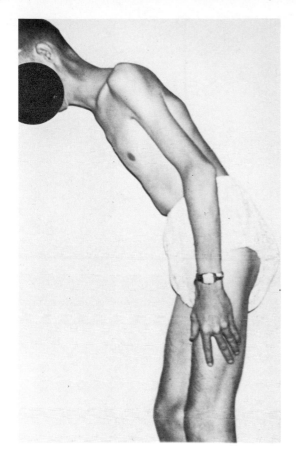

Figure 3-19.
Marie-Strümpell
arthritis of the
spine.

boo spine (Fig. 3-20). Ankylosis of the hip joints is common, with the knees being affected less frequently.

Clinical Findings. The bony bridging of the spine and ankylosis of the hips result in a so-called poker spine, with rigidity, increased dorsal kyphosis, loss of lumbar lordosis, and pain and limitation of motion of the hips. The sacro-iliac is often the first joint involved.

Treatment. Treatment includes exercises, positioning, and bracing in an attempt to prevent the severe flexion deformities of the spine. Occasionally, osteotomy of the spine and arthroplasty of the hips are indicated to improve function.

Bursitis

Bursitis is an inflammation of the sac (bursa) covering a bony prominence. Often the underlying tendons may be inflamed, in which case *tendinitis* is combined with bursitis.

Cause. The cause may be traumatic, infectious, or idiopathic.

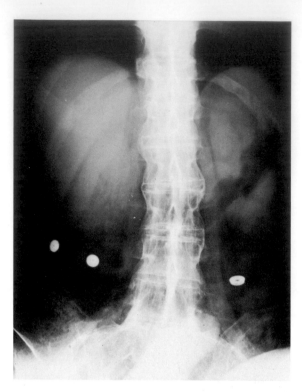

Figure 3-20. X-ray of a so-called bamboo spine.

Figure 3-21. Ole-cranon bursitis in the right arm.

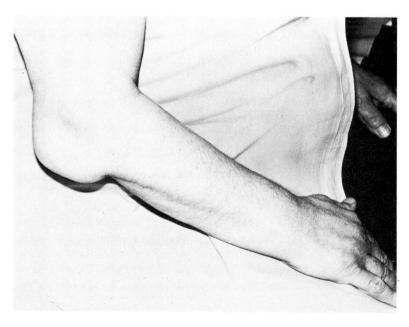

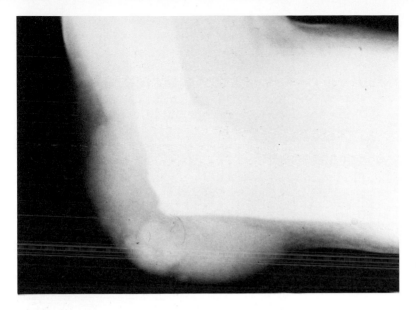

Figure 3-22. X-ray of olecranon bursitis. Note the soft tissue swelling and calcification.

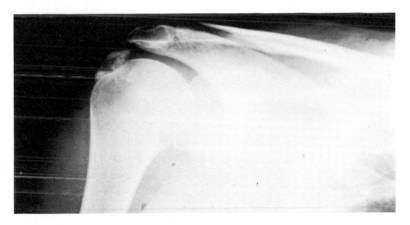

Figure 3-23. Calcific tendinitis and bursitis of the right shoulder.

Clinical Findings. Acute pain in the shoulder without injury, causing inability to abduct the arm, is the most common manifestation of subacromial bursitis and rotator cuff tendinitis. Other common bursitic problems are olecranon bursitis, with the so-called goose-egg appearance of the olecranon bursa beneath the skin (Fig. 3-21), prepatellar bursitis of the knee, often called housemaid's knee, and bursitis or tendinitis of the extensor origin at the elbow, known as tennis elbow.

X-ray Findings. Calcium may or may not be present in the tendons just beneath the bursa (Figs. 3-22, 3-23).

Treatment. Resting the joint and administering antiinflammatory and pain-relieving drugs may suffice. On the other hand, in a case of severe acute bursitis and tendinitis, local injection with an anesthetic and corticosteroids often gives dramatic and immediate relief. Occasionally, in cases of shoulder bursitis that cannot be managed conservatively, incision of the underlying edematous and often calcific area will be necessary; this procedure usually gives dramatic relief. Incision of the tendon sheath may be necessary in de Quervain's disease, which is tenosynovitis affecting the long abductor and the short extensor to the thumb and their common tendon sheath at the radial styloid process.

Myositis

Myositis is an inflammation of a muscle or muscles. Gas gangrene is a form of myositis.

Cause. It may be caused by trauma (contusion), infection, or systemic disease.

Clinical Findings. Clinical manifestations depend on the cause and intensity of muscular involvement.

Treatment. Treatment also depends on the underlying cause, and ranges from supportive and conservative management to surgical intervention.

Myositis Ossificans

Myositis ossificans is the formation of bone in a traumatized muscle (Fig. 3-24).

Cause. The muscle is traumatized adjacent to bone and hemorrhage occurs. Occasionally, similar conditions develop around the joint after burns and after neurologic diseases without trauma.

Pathology. The pathological process is not clearly understood, but is thought to be some type of metaplasia of connective tissue elements and fibroblasts, with the production of new bone.

Clinical Findings. This condition is found most frequently in the quadriceps muscle of the thigh and the brachialis muscle of the arm. There is some discoloration and swelling from hematoma after injury, and the extremity has a firm, brawny appearance with marked limitation of motion that does not respond to forceful manipulation and physical therapy. Flexion contractures of the joints may occur secondary to the new bone formation.

Treatment. Usually, with very gentle exercises and time, the new bone matures and good function returns; however, surgical excision is necessary in some cases.

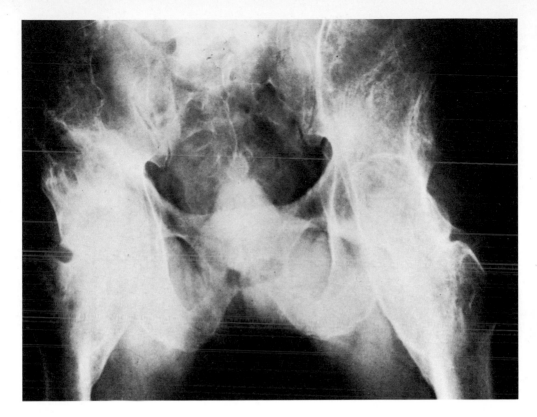

Figure 3-24. Myositis ossificans of both hips in a patient with traumatic paraplegia.

NEOPLASTIC DISORDERS

The tissues of the skeletal system may undergo tumor formation, with tumors arising either primarily from the skeletal system or as metastases to the skeletal system from other sites. Primary bone tumors may be benign (Fig. 3-25) or malignant. Malignant bone tumors grow rapidly, are hard to diagnose early, and are frequently fatal. Metastatic disease to the bone is most often from sites in the breast, prostate, kidney, thyroid, or lung.

Osteochondroma

An osteochondroma is a benign tumor composed of bone covered by a cartilaginous cap (Fig. 3-26).

Clinical Findings. It is usually seen in growing children and is manifested by a firm, nontender, painless swelling near a joint. These tumors are most commonly found in the distal femur or proximal tibia. Because of their prominence, the area may be subject to trauma and discomfort.

Treatment. If it is large and subject to repeated trauma, an osteochondroma is surgically removed.

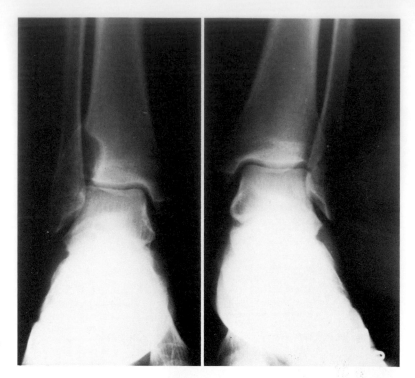

Figure 3-25. Benign tumor of the right ankle. This was an aneurysmal bone cyst.

Figure 3-26. Osteochondroma of the distal right femur.

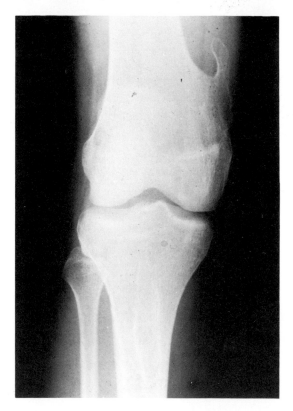

Chondroma or Enchondroma

A chondroma, or enchondroma, is a benign tumor occurring in a central location in a bone, usually a phalange or the humerus. It has a potential for undergoing malignant transformation, particularly when situated in a long bone or the pelvis.

Clinical Findings. It is usually not seen unless it is detected by x-ray or causes a pathological fracture.

Treatment. Usually no treatment is indicated unless pathological fracture, evidence of enlargement, or symptoms occur, in which case one has to suspect malignant transformation.

Osteoid-Osteoma

Osteoid-osteoma is a small rarefying bone lesion composed of vascular fibrous tissue, fibroblasts, and spicules of newly formed osteoid.

Clinical Findings. Usually seen in young adults in the tibia and femur, it is characterized by an aching pain in the affected extremity, usually dramatically relieved by aspirin. X-rays show sclerosis of the bone around a radiolucent nidus.

Treatment. Surgical excision of the nidus gives relief.

Osteogenic Sarcoma

Osteogenic sarcoma is a rapidly developing malignant tumor of the bone, with characteristic production of new bone (Fig. 3-27).

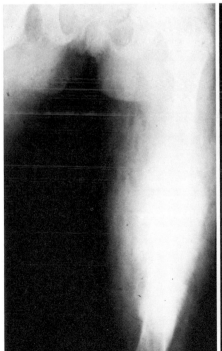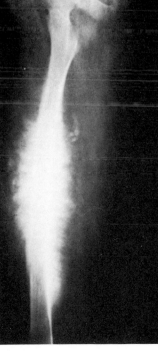

Figure 3-27. Osteogenic sarcoma of the left femur with new bone formation.

Clinical Findings. Most commonly seen in young people between the ages of 10 and 20 years, it occurs in the long bones at the most rapidly growing areas: distal femur, proximal tibia, proximal humerus, and proximal femur. The patient will develop aching discomfort, swelling, and pain that is rapidly progressive. X-rays show destruction of the bone, with new bone formation occurring at the same time.

Treatment. Amputation, with chemotherapy, is necessary.

Giant-Cell Tumor

Giant-cell tumor is an osteolytic tumor occurring in young adults at the end of a long bone (epiphyseal area), and is typified by an abundance of characteristic giant cells (Fig. 3-28).

Clinical Findings. This tumor occurs after the epiphyseal plate is ossified and growth is completed, and is most commonly seen in young adults between the ages of 15 and 35 years in the epiphyses of the distal femur, the distal radius, and the proximal tibia. The patient has constant, progressive pain with swelling, limitation of joint motion, and finally pathological fracture.

Treatment. Excision is done if possible; otherwise, curettage and bone grafting are done. Recurrence and malignant changes do occur.

Figure 3-28. Giant-cell tumor of the proximal right tibia.

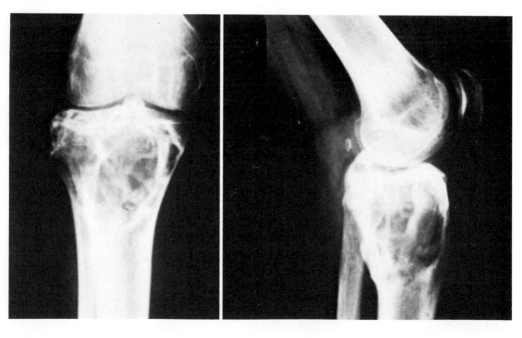

Unicameral Bone Cyst

Unicameral bone cyst is a cystic lesion that occurs in a long bone (Fig. 3-29), usually in children.

Clinical Findings. There may be no symptoms. Often the cyst is detected when the arm is fractured with minor trauma.

Treatment. Excision and bone grafting are done. Occasionally a bone cyst will heal after fracture.

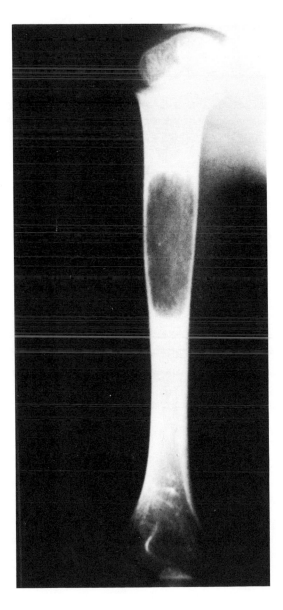

Figure 3-29. Unicameral bone cyst in the right humerus.

Fibrous Dysplasia

Fibrous dysplasia is a condition of unknown cause characterized by fibrous tissue replacement of the skeleton. It may be monostotic (one bone) (Fig. 3-30) or polyostotic (multiple bones).

Clinical Findings. Dysplasia usually starts in early childhood but is usually mild and asymptomatic. It may be discovered by x-ray when symptoms have developed, or the deformity of one of the long bones may become apparent at a later age. Pathological fractures occur, and there is frequently asymmetry of the head and face with characteristic large, brown, irregular patches of skin pigmentation, particularly with the polyostotic form of the disease. The clinical course is ex-

Figure 3-30. Monostotic fibrous dysplasia of the right tibia.

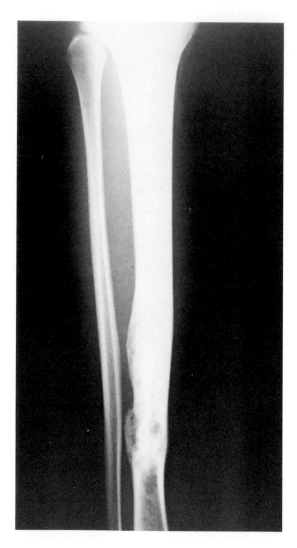

tremely variable. The diagnosis is made by examination of biopsy material.

Treatment. The deformity is often severe when the fibrous dysplasia develops early in life, and corrective surgery may be necessary.

Multiple Myeloma

Multiple myeloma is a neoplasm consisting basically of cells resembling plasma cells, which characteristically invade and replace cancellous bone slowly in older individuals (Fig. 3-31). Patients with this disease are usually between the ages of 40 and 60 years.

Clinical Findings. Affected individuals have gradually increasing pain, often vague at first, frequently in the spine and chest. Pathological fractures may develop, and compression fractures of the spine are commonly seen, with generalized decreased bone mass (osteopenia). Characteristic laboratory findings include the presence of Bence Jones protein in the urine, an altered albumin-globulin ratio, anemia, and a characteristic electrophoretic serum pattern.

Treatment. Treatment is essentially palliative. Radiation therapy is used.

Figure 3-31. Multiple myeloma (punched-out lesions).

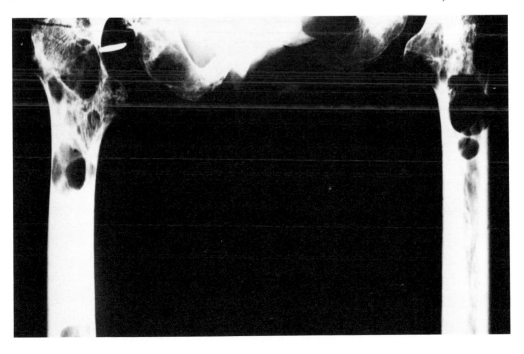

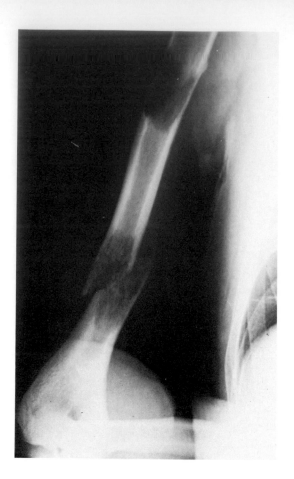

Figure 3-32. Metastatic bone disease with pathological fracture of the humerus.

Metastatic Bone Disease

Metastatic bone disease is seen most commonly when the primary tumor site is in the breast, kidney, thyroid, prostate, or lung.

Clinical Findings. Metastases do not usually occur below the elbows and knees. Pain, pathological fractures of the spine and long bones, and anemia are seen (Fig. 3-32).

Treatment. The treatment of metastatic bone disease is primarily medication to relieve pain and reduce discomfort. Radiation therapy is occasionally used to control pain. Often internal fixation and intramedullary nailing is of great benefit prophylactically or after pathological fracture. Prosthetic replacement for metastatic disease localized to the head and neck of the femur is also beneficial.

Paget's Disease (Osteitis Deformans)

Paget's disease (osteitis deformans) is a common chronic affection of the skeleton that occurs in individuals past middle

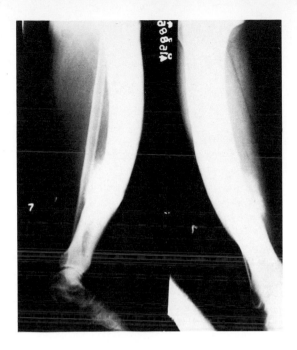

Figure 3-33. Paget's disease of the right tibia.

age and is characterized by thickening and deformity of bony structures and by complications of fractures and malignant degeneration (Fig. 3-33). The cause is unknown. Men are affected more often than women, and the disease is usually seen after the age of 50 years. It is characterized by a process of extensive osteoclastic destruction accompanied by increased vascularity and fibrosis with new bone formation. The process is disorganized and the bone is not of normal strength.

Clinical Findings. Often the patient's skull size will expand (individual finds that a larger hat is needed). Commonly there is progressive deformity of the tibia with thickening of the bone and bowing anterolaterally. The disease is often diagnosed by x-ray examination. Calcium and phosphorus levels are normal, but the alkaline phosphate determination is higher in Paget's disease than in any other condition; its level is an index of bone formation.

Treatment. Immobilization reverses the stress stimulus for bone formation, but because of the disease bone destruction continues. This can cause a dangerous hypercalcemia, which must be watched for and controlled when a patient with Paget's disease has to be relatively immobilized for any reason. Osteotomy is performed for deformity of bone, when indicated, and internal fixation of fractures is done to minimize the necessity for immobilization.

METABOLIC DISEASES

Gout

Gout is a hereditary condition of disturbed uric acid metabolism.

Pathology. Serum uric acid is elevated and urate salts are deposited in articular, periarticular, and subcutaneous tissues in attacks of acute arthritis. Gout is most common in men around the age of 40 years.

Clinical Findings. The patient has recurrent attacks of acute arthritis, with redness, pain, and extreme sensitivity of the skin about the involved joint. The metatarsophalangeal joint of the great toe is most commonly affected. Laboratory studies reveal an elevated serum uric acid.

Treatment. Immobilization and ice packs to the joint may help; occasionally, moist hot compresses offer more relief. The pain can be severe and narcotics may be required. Colchicine is a specific drug for this condition. Phenylbutazone is also an effective therapeutic agent.

Osteoporosis

Osteoporosis is manifested by a diffuse reduction in bone density (osteopenia).

Cause. There is decreased formation of a protein matrix in which calcium is deposited. It is not a problem of calcium metabolism, but one of protein metabolism. Osteoporosis is seen most commonly in elderly women.

Pathology. The decreasing stress factor, which normally stimulates protein and osteoid formation, and hormonal changes are important factors. The bones are not of normal strength due to the diminution in protein matrix and resultant decreased bone mass.

Clinical Findings. Compression fractures of the spine with minor trauma are common. Hip fractures, Colles' fractures, and fractures of the surgical neck of the humerus often occur when these patients fall.

Treatment. Treatment is essentially symptomatic. Simple exercises and activities tend to promote osteoid formation. Administration of hormones may be beneficial.

Osteomalacia

Osteomalacia is decreased bone mass (osteopenia) caused by abnormalities of calcium metabolism.

Cause. Osteomalacia can be caused by anything that interferes with and lowers the serum calcium. Rickets is a form of osteomalacia that may occur in childhood.

Pathology. The protein matrix of bone is formed normally but the calcification process does not occur as it should.

Clinical Findings. Symptoms are related to the causative

factors, deformities of the weight bearing structures, and generalized skeletal pain and tenderness.

Treatment. Both calcium and vitamin D are given orally and a diet high in protein is instituted. Those disorders interfering with calcium absorption are corrected. Osteotomies may be necessary to correct deformities.

INFECTION OF BONE

Osteomyelitis

Osteomyelitis literally means inflammation of bone and its marrow regardless of cause; however, by common usage it is applied to an infection by pyogenic bacteria.

ACUTE OSTEOMYELITIS. Acute osteomyelitis is a rapidly destructive pyogenic infection, usually hematogenous in origin, occurring most often in infants and children (Fig. 3-34). It usually starts in a metaphysis of an actively growing long bone.

Cause. It occurs most commonly in infancy and childhood, probably by introduction of bacteria into the bone through a blood vessel.

Pathology. In a growing child the most vascularized area is in the metaphysis adjacent to the epiphyseal plate. The infected embolus contains organisms, and an inflammatory reac-

Figure 3-34. Findings after bone destruction in the left hip from acute osteomyelitis in infancy.

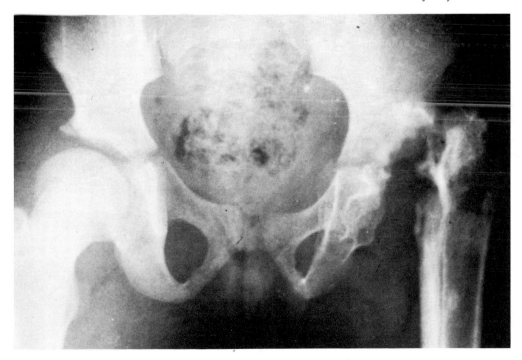

tion occurs in the bone, producing exudate, hyperemia, and severe pain.

Clinical Findings. The child is usually obviously ill, with a high fever, high white cell count, a very sensitive extremity, and tenderness in a limb which he or she will not move.

Treatment. Treatment consists of antibiotics, supportive therapy, and drainage of the area by windowing the bone. Topical antibiotics may also be useful.

CHRONIC OSTEOMYELITIS. Chronic osteomyelitis is a low-grade pyogenic infection that may persist for months or years after subsidence of the original acute bone infection.

Clinical Findings. The patient often has episodes of recurrent drainage and flare-up of acute symptoms. As the bone

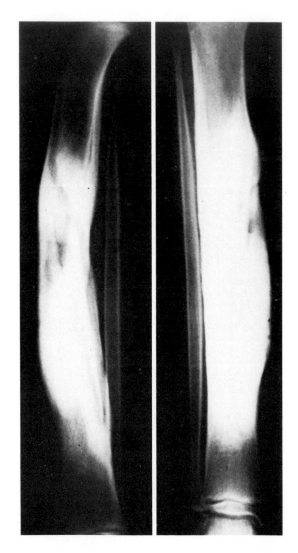

Figure 3-35. Chronic osteomyelitis of the right tibia with sequestrum. Note the dense, white, dead bone.

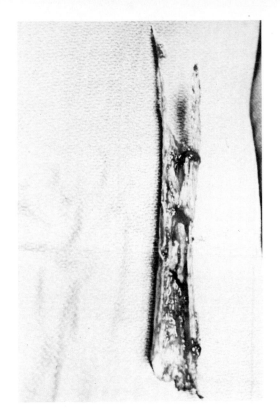

Figure 3-36.
Removed
sequestrum.

attempts to eradicate the infection, necrotic cortical bone may be retained as a sequestrum (Fig. 3-35). This continues to act as a foreign body and may have to be surgically removed before the drainage will cease, or the sequestrum may be discharged spontaneously. As the bone heals around the area of chronic osteomyelitis the bone will thicken and become sclerotic. There are often chronic changes in the skin overlying an area of chronic osteomyelitis.

Treatment. Often a sequestrectomy and removal of portions of the involved bone is necessary (Fig. 3-36). It is difficult to eradicate an area of chronic osteomyelitis. Pathological fracture can develop if too radical a bone débridement is done. Amputation may even be necessary.

DEGENERATIVE JOINT DISEASE

Osteoarthritis

Osteoarthritis is a degenerative process which affects the articular cartilage chiefly in weight bearing joints, giving rise to symptoms of pain and stiffness. Some degenerative changes in the joints occur as a normal process of aging. The degree and effect on the individual vary.

Pathology. There is atrophy and degeneration of the articular cartilage with softening, adjacent sclerosis, and spur formation of the subchondral bone. The joint space narrows due to the gradual loss of cartilage (Fig. 3-37).

Clinical Findings. Most people over the age of 50 years will show x-ray evidence of some osteoarthritis, but only a small number of these individuals will have significant joint symptoms. There are no constitutional manifestations related to this disorder. The patient has pain and stiffness, particularly in the morning and after sitting in one position for any length of time. Often comfort improves with motion initially, but after prolonged activity symptoms increasingly develop. In the hand, the joint involvement is the opposite of that in rheumatoid arthritis. The distal interphalangeal (DIP) joints are usually involved (Heberden's nodes).

Treatment. Conservative measures include exercises to maintain range of motion and improve muscle strength, use of heat, and administration of anti-inflammatory drugs. Weight loss relieves the constant strain on the weight bearing

Figure 3-37. Osteoarthritis of the left hip. Note the loss of articular space.

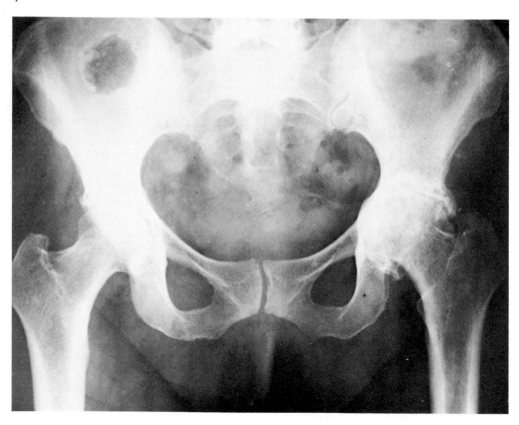

joints, and if the patient is obese this measure is in order. Surgery is very helpful in management of severe pain and disability from degenerative arthritis. Included in surgical management are arthroplasty of the joint as well as osteotomy to relieve stresses and strains on the joint; occasionally, fusion of an involved joint is helpful. Total joint replacement for osteoarthritis of the hip and knee has become increasingly popular in recent years and gives excellent results.

Traumatic Arthritis

Traumatic arthritis is a loss of articular cartilage with roughening and malfunction of a joint developing secondary to previous injury to the cartilaginous surface of the joint (Fig. 3-38).

Clinical Findings. Traumatic arthritis can occur in a joint previously damaged by trauma, infection, excessive use, or maldevelopment. The incongruities of the articular surfaces lead to gradually increasing wear and tear with age and use.

Figure 3-38. Traumatic arthritis of both hips secondary to childhood dysplasia.

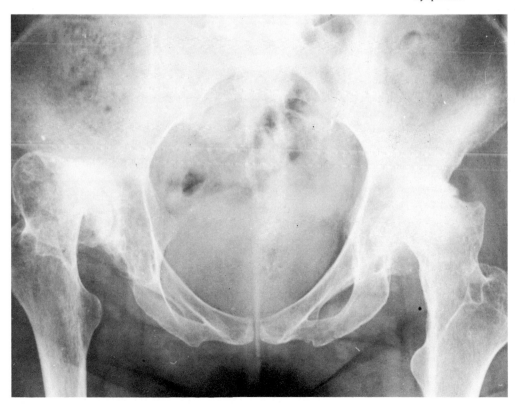

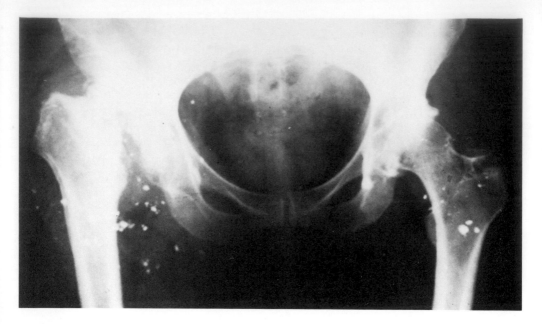

*Figure 3-39. Char-
cot disease of
right hip.*

The late findings in any one joint are indistinct from osteoarthritis (degenerative arthritis).

Treatment. Treatment is basically the same as for degenerative arthritis.

Charcot Joint

Charcot joint is a form of chronic, progressive degenerative
arthropathy affecting one or more peripheral or spinal joints
(Figs. 3-39, 3-40).

Cause. It is a complication of various neurologic disorders
such as tabes dorsalis of syphilitic origin, diabetic neuropathy,
myelomeningocele, and spinal cord compression.

Pathology. The joint loses its normal proprioception and
pain sensation. The normal reflex mechanisms by which the
joint tends to protect itself from excessive stresses and strains
function poorly. The result is an unstable and severely degen-
erated joint.

Clinical Findings. The patient is usually a man over 40 years
old. Several joints are frequently involved. The amount of
discomfort is milder than the dramatic clinical and x-ray
appearance of the joint suggests.

X-ray Findings. On x-rays this condition is similar to exag-
gerated osteoarthritis. Intra-articular fractures and loose
bodies in the joint are common.

Treatment. The joint is immobilized, with restricted weight
bearing. If an effusion is present it may be aspirated to relieve

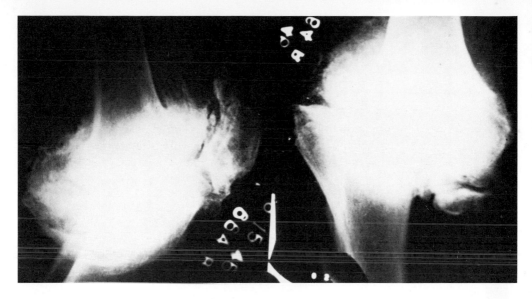

Figure 3-40. Charcot disease of right knee.

the joint distension. Surgery is usually restricted to amputation or arthrodesis due to the poor tolerance of the joint to surgery. Fusion of major weight bearing joints may be done; however, a successful fusion is difficult to achieve and nonunion is common.

Hemophilic Arthritis

Hemophilic arthritis consists of degenerative changes of the bone and cartilage of a joint associated with marked fibrous tissue contractures.

Cause. Repeated joint hemorrhages in the patient with hemophilia are the etiological factor. This disorder is most frequently seen in the knees and elbows.

Treatment. Prophylactic treatment consists of avoidance of trauma. In the presence of acute hemarthrosis the joint is immobilized by a cast or a splint. Further bleeding is controlled by the use of whole blood or plasma. Restoration of joint motion after bleeding has subsided is accomplished by gradual active exercises. Surgery in these patients is avoided if at all possible. Identification of the abnormal blood factor and its maintenance replacement has resulted in improved prophylaxis of the ravages of this disease and has allowed orthopedic surgery to be carried out when necessary.

NEUROMUSCULAR DISORDERS

Neuromuscular disorders that affect the musculoskeletal system and give rise to orthopedic conditions may be of congenital, infectious, metabolic, traumatic, or unknown origin. The manifestations of the disorder will depend primarily on the level of involvement of the neuromuscular system

Any involvement of the spinal cord above the level of the anterior horn cells and peripheral nerves represents an upper motor-neuron lesion. Upper motor-neuron lesions are characterized by the development of muscular spasticity, hyperreflexia, and pathological reflexes such as the Babinski sign (great toe goes up when the plantar surface of the foot is stroked). Cerebral palsy is an example of an upper motor-neuron lesion.

If the anterior horn cells, cauda equina, peripheral nerves, or plexuses are involved, the condition is called a lower motor-neuron lesion. It is characterized by flaccidity of the muscles, absent tendon reflexes, muscular atrophy, and a reaction of degeneration. Poliomyelitis and nerve root compression syndrome are examples of lower motor-neuron lesions.

There may be a failure of muscle function due to a problem intrinsic to the muscle itself, such as progressive muscular dystrophy, or due to some type of interference with the neural transition of impulses at the myoneural junction, such as myasthenia gravis.

Cerebral Palsy

Cerebral palsy is a state of muscle dysfunction caused by damage to or defect of the upper motor neurons either in the brain stem or in the brain. Such damage results in interference with voluntary motor function.

Cause. Causes are multiple and may arise during or after birth. Congenital defective brain development and cerebral anoxia at the time of birth can cause cerebral palsy, as can encephalitis and trauma after birth.

Clinical Findings. There are several types of cerebral palsy manifested by spasticity, athetoid motions, or ataxia, and there are also mixed types of cerebral palsy.

Treatment. Treatment requires all of the resources of the rehabilitation team. The ultimate improvement of the patient requires attention to speech difficulties and mental problems as well as to orthopedic and musculoskeletal problems. Orthopedic surgery is of the greatest benefit in spastic cerebral palsy. Overactive muscles can be lengthened or transplanted, muscle spasms can be reduced by neurectomy, and bone surgery can be undertaken to counteract the skeletal effects of long-term muscle imbalance secondary to spasticity. Spastic paralysis may occur in the adult secondary to a cerebrovascular accident; the adult requires muscle reeducation, appropriate splints and exercises to prevent contractures, and the use of braces. Occasionally muscle and tendon transplants are indicated.

Anterior Poliomyelitis

Anterior poliomyelitis (infantile paralysis) is essentially a disease of childhood in which the anterior horn cell in the cord is affected, producing a flaccid paralysis. It is usually asymmetric and sensory nerves are not involved. Fortunately, this disease has become increasingly rare in the United States.

Treatment. Supportive care and maintenance of comfort are needed, along with prevention of contractures during the acute stage and reeducation and strengthening of nonparalyzed muscle groups in the convalescent stage. Numerous orthopedic surgical procedures are helpful in the residual stage, including tendon and muscle transplants, arthrodesis of unstable joints, epiphyseal arrest, and operations to equalize leg lengths.

Friedreich's Ataxia

Friedreich's ataxia is a degenerative disease involving chiefly the posterior columns of the spinal cord. It affects children and young adults and produces an ataxic, uncoordinated gait and often a cavus or claw foot which requires surgical alignment to improve weight bearing.

Charcot-Marie-Tooth Disease

Charcot-Marie-Tooth disease is a familial neurologic disease of unknown cause associated with degenerative changes of the spinal roots and the peripheral nerves in the posterior columns of the spinal cord. Usually the peripheral nerve is affected with a drop-foot deformity, which may require surgery of the foot (triple arthrodesis) as well as muscle and tendon transplants.

Obstetrical Palsy

Obstetrical palsy is the name given to a traction injury to the infant's brachial plexus caused by pulling on the arm during a difficult delivery.

Pathology. The most common injury involves the upper brachial plexus nerve roots (5 and 6) and is characterized by paralysis involving mainly the external rotators and the abductors of the upper arm and shoulder.

Clinical Findings. The arm lies in the internally rotated, adducted position, and the child cannot abduct the arm (Erb's palsy).

Treatment. Range of motion exercises to prevent contractures are in order, and usually spontaneous recovery occurs. If it does not, sometimes muscle releases or osteotomies improve function.

Polyneuritis

Polyneuritis is a term which may be applied to any condition associated with the irritation of multiple peripheral nerves.

Cause. Nutritional causes such as avitaminosis and alcoholism may be implicated. Diabetes is a frequent metabolic cause, and lead poisoning may also produce peripheral neuritis.

Clinical Findings. Pain and tenderness along the nerve with paresthesias and partial or complete paralysis of the muscles affected by the nerve may be present.

Infectious Polyneuritis

Infectious polyneuritis (Guillain-Barré syndrome) is an acute ascending progressive symmetric paralysis, usually following an upper respiratory tract infection. It differs from poliomyelitis in that it is almost always very symmetric, the patient is usually afebrile, and there is an abnormal, elevated spinal fluid protein content. Spontaneous recovery usually occurs.

Progressive Muscular Dystrophy

Progressive muscular dystrophy is a degenerative disease of muscle tissue of unknown etiology.

Clinical Findings. The disease is usually seen during the first 3 years of life. It affects the shoulder girdle and pelvic girdle primarily, with progressive weakness over a period of months and years and the development of contractures, deformity, and general debility. There is an increased excretion of creatine and a decreased excretion of creatinine in the urine.

Treatment. There is no known treatment.

Myasthenia Gravis

Myasthenia gravis is a disease characterized by excessive fatigability of voluntary muscles.

Cause. The disease may be due to an abnormality at the myoneural junction.

Pathology. Myasthenia gravis may affect a single muscle, a muscle group, or all muscles. Females are more commonly affected than males.

Clinical Findings. Muscle fatigue and weakness are aggravated by exertion and muscle strength is restored by rest. Usually facial muscle symptoms are noted first.

Treatment. Administration of neostigmine bromide, a parasympathetic stimulant, reverses the manifestations, and treatment is accomplished by administering properly adjusted dosages.

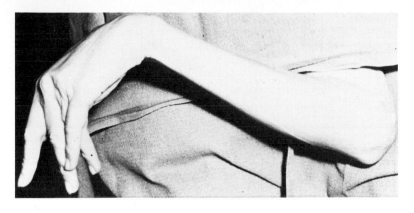

Figure 3-41. A wrist with radial nerve palsy.

Trauma to Peripheral Nerves

Certain peripheral nerves are subjected to trauma more frequently than others.

The *radial nerve* is damaged in association with fractures of the midshaft of the humerus. The patient is unable to actively raise the wrist, the thumb, and the metacarpophalangeal joints of the hand (Fig. 3-41).

The *median nerve* may be involved in the carpal tunnel syndrome or be damaged by a dislocation of the lunate bone at the wrist. The patient is unable to actively oppose the thumb to the fingers.

The *ulnar nerve* may be damaged by trauma or fracture involving the medial epicondyle of the humerus. The patient may be unable to spread and bring together all of the fingers. Clawing of the fourth and fifth digits may develop.

The *sciatic nerve* may be damaged by the femoral head following a traumatic posterior dislocation of the hip or in association with a fracture through the midshaft of the femur. The patient may have complete paralysis of all the muscles of the lower leg and foot and partial paralysis of the thigh muscles.

The *axillary nerve* may be damaged in association with an anteriorly dislocated shoulder joint. The patient may be unable to actively abduct the arm at the shoulder joint.

The *common peroneal nerve* may be damaged by excessive pressure or injury to the head and neck of the fibula. The patient may be unable to actively dorsiflex or evert the foot (foot drop). The first sign may be inability to dorsiflex the great toe.

Herniated Intervertebral Disc

Herniated intervertebral disc is the rupture or herniation of the nucleus pulposus (the center of the intervertebral disc) into the posterior longitudinal spinal ligament or spinal canal, causing pressure on the adjacent spinal nerve root as it passes on its way to exit from the spine.

Cause. Ordinarily the nucleus pulposus is maintained in place by a thick fibrous band called the annulus fibrosus; a rupture occurs when this wall has weakened or is torn because of attritional or degenerative changes.

Clinical Findings. A herniated intervertebral disc of the lumbosacral region is seen most commonly in men between the ages of 20 and 45 years. The individual may complain of back pain, with radiation over the course of the sciatic nerve or with leg pain alone. So-called sciatic scoliosis is frequently seen in the acute condition. Bending, lifting, coughing, and sneezing will aggravate the leg pain. Tenderness over the affected vertebral interspace and the course of the sciatic nerve may or may not be present. Straight leg raising is positive. The patient may complain of a sensation of numbness and tingling in the toes and feet. The Achilles reflex may be depressed or absent. Herniation is most common in the discs of the interspaces of the fourth and fifth lumbar vertebrae and the fifth lumbar and first sacral vertebrae. In the presence of a cervical nerve root compression secondary to a herniated disc the individual usually complains of shoulder and arm pain associated with numbness and tingling in the hand and fingers; the pain usually radiates from the shoulder and arm into the forearm and fingers. Coughing, sneezing, or straining, as well as jarring the neck or applying pressure to the top of the head, will increase the pain. The level of nerve root involvement determines the objective signs. The most common areas of involvement are the interspaces of the fifth and sixth and the sixth and seventh cervical vertebrae.

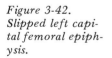
Figure 3-42. Slipped left capital femoral epiphysis.

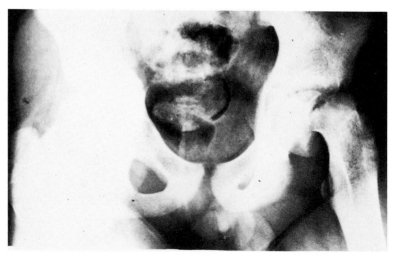

Treatment. Conservative management usually suffices. This consists of bed rest, traction, muscle relaxants, analgesics, and local heat. A supportive back brace or corset is also used in some cases. Unrelenting, unmanageable pain and a progressive neurologic deficit may make surgical excision of the protruded disc material advisable.

DISORDERS OF THE EPIPHYSES
Slipped Capital Femoral Epiphysis
Slipped capital femoral epiphysis is the displacement of the capital femoral epiphysis in a downward and backward position from the femoral neck (Fig. 3-42).

Cause. This disorder occurs most frequently in boys from 10 to 16 years old and may be bilateral. It occurs most frequently in the overweight child with underdeveloped genitalia or the tall thin child undergoing a rapid adolescent growth spurt. The cause is not clearly understood.

Clinical Findings. The patient commonly complains of some vague discomfort about the hip with radiation of pain to the knee. A limp is usually seen. There is a limited range of motion of the extremity with shortening and limitation of internal rotation. Occasionally the displacement of the epiphysis may follow a specific episode of trauma to the hip.

X-ray Findings. The actual slipping of the capital femoral epiphysis is first noted on the lateral x-ray. The epiphysis tends to displace downward and backward in relation to the femoral neck. The condition is frequently hard to see on an anteroposterior x-ray.

Treatment. Surgical intervention is necessary for internal fixation of the slipped capital femoral epiphysis. Frequently this may be accomplished without reduction; however, in severe cases reduction and internal fixation is necessary (Fig. 3-43). Residual deformity of the head and neck of the femur

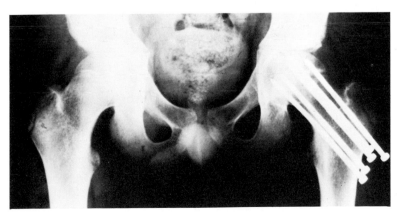

Figure 3-43. Reduction and internal fixation of slipped capital femoral epiphysis.

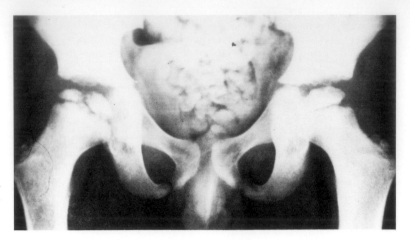

Figure 3-44. Legg-Calvé-Perthes' disease of the right hip.

may cause the complication of degenerative arthritis in later years.

Legg-Calvé-Perthes' Disease

Legg-Calvé-Perthes' disease is avascular necrosis of the capital femoral epiphysis occurring in childhood (Fig. 3-44). Its etiology is unknown.

Pathology. Massive necrosis of the bone of the capital femoral epiphysis occurs secondary to avascular necrosis. The condition is self-limiting in that bone repair begins almost immediately following the necrosis. Complete healing does occur, but the contour of the epiphysis may be flattened and it never regains a completely normal shape and appearance. This condition may lead to serious hip disability later in life.

Clinical Findings. This disease is seen most commonly in boys between the ages of 3 and 12 years. It is usually unilateral but may be bilateral. The child usually has discomfort in the hip area with referred knee pain. He also has an antalgic gait. There is limitation of hip motion, and spasm of the adductor muscles may be present.

X-ray Findings. In the early stages the epiphysis appears to be thin or flattened; later it seems to be fragmented. It then coalesces into a single mass of healing bone as repair proceeds, and the femoral neck tends to shorten and broaden.

Treatment. A variety of conservative as well as surgical treatments are used. In general, conservative management consists of either non-weight bearing or weight bearing in an abduction brace. Surgical treatment may be an osteotomy to place the femoral head in an abducted weight bearing position. The principle of treatment, whether by bracing or surgery, is to contain the femoral head deep in the socket (an abducted position accomplishes this) while it undergoes its healing phase. The normal acetabulum tends to keep the femoral head molded in a round shape rather than letting it flatten and deform.

Osgood-Schlatter Disease
Osgood-Schlatter disease is osteochondritis of the tibial spine apophysis.

Cause. It is thought by some to be of traumatic origin secondary to repeated flexion of the knee against a tight quadriceps, particularly during the rapid growth period. Boys are particularly predisposed to this condition.

Clinical Findings. Any activity which requires strong quadriceps contraction and therefore strain on the tubercle causes pain. Extension of the knee against resistance is also painful.

X-ray Findings. X-rays may show some fragmentation and separation of the tibial tubercle.

Treatment. Symptomatic treatment of this condition consists of restriction of activities, or immobilization of the extremity if the patient is experiencing severe pain. The disease is usually self-limited.

Sever's Disease
Sever's disease is osteochondritis of the apophysis of the os calcis that occurs during the rapid growth period.

Cause. This condition is seen more frequently in boys than in girls and is thought to have a traumatic onset due to pull of the Achilles tendon on the apophysis of the heel.

Clinical Findings. There is pain in the heel which is aggravated by walking and especially by running, with a resultant limp. The back of the heel is locally tender.

X-ray Findings. X-rays may show fragmentation of the apophysis of the os calcis but are usually normal.

Treatment. The treatment is symptomatic. An elastic bandage wrap may be used; crutches are sometimes required for relief of pain.

CONDITIONS NOT OTHERWISE CLASSIFIED
Avascular (Aseptic) Necrosis of the Hip
Avascular or aseptic necrosis of the femoral head of the hip is death of bony tissue in the head of the femur. If it occurs in childhood it is known as Legg-Calvé-Perthes' disease.

Cause. Interruption of the circulation to an area of bone results in death of that segment of bone tissue. It may occur secondary to a fracture of the neck of the femur or a dislocated hip. It is often seen in patients who require long-term steroid therapy (for example, a patient with a kidney trans-

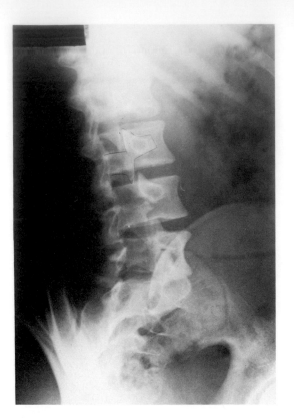

Figure 3-45. Oblique x-ray of the lumbar spine. Note the similarity to a scottie dog outlined on the third lumbar vertebra with a defect in the collar at the fourth lumbar vertebra.

plant), and alcoholics show an increased incidence of this problem. In most cases the cause is unknown.

Clinical Findings. Pain may first be noted in the thigh or knee, with an associated slight limp. The hip is painful following long periods of weight bearing or after sitting for long periods of time. Over a period of from a few months to several years, hip motion becomes progressively restricted in all directions.

Treatment. Long-term protection of the joint with a cane or crutches combined with mild analgesics is in order. Weight loss helps if the patient is overweight. If deformity of the joint and disabling arthritis occur, total hip arthroplasty may be required.

Spondylolysis

Spondylolysis is the term used to describe a defect in the posterior arch of the vertebral body when forward slipping has not occurred.

Cause. It is thought to be of congenital or traumatic origin.

Clinical Findings. Patients usually complain of low back pain which becomes progressively worse. Gradually symptoms of nerve root irritation develop.

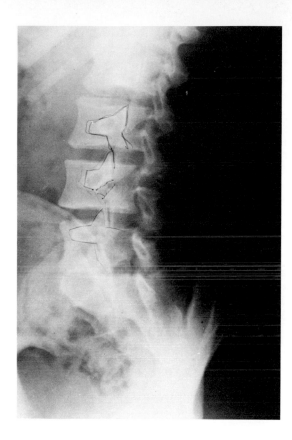

Figure 3-46.
Oblique view of
spondylolysis of
the lumbar spine.
Note the scottie
dog outlined in
ink with a collar
defect at the
fourth lumbar
vertebra.

X-ray Findings. A defect in the pars interarticularis is seen
on the oblique views (Figs. 3-45, 3-46). This is known as the
collar on the scottie dog. The anteroposterior and lateral
views may not show the defect. The levels most often involved are the fourth and fifth lumbar vertebrae.

Spondylolisthesis
Spondylolisthesis is the forward slipping of a vertebra on the
vertebral body below it secondary to a pars interarticularis
defect (spondylolysis).
  Cause. Some authorities believe this to be a congenital developmental condition while others think it is traumatic in
origin.
  Clinical Findings. Patients usually complain of low back
pain which becomes progressively worse. Gradual symptoms
of nerve root irritation develop, as shown by decreased
straight leg raising.
  X-ray Findings. A lateral spot x-ray reveals forward displacement of the vertebral body on the body below. Oblique
x-rays show a pars interarticularis defect (collar on the scottie dog).

Treatment. Conservative management including rest, restriction of activities, and the use of a back support is instituted. Surgical intervention may be necessary if disability is progressive and pain is severe and persistent. Spinal fusion is the surgical procedure usually performed.

Baker's Cyst (Popliteal Cyst)
Baker's cyst (popliteal cyst) is a firm, tense cystic mass occasionally found along the medial border of the popliteal space.

Cause. The etiology is often unknown. Many feel that these cysts are secondary to synovial disease, irritation of the knee joint, or inflammation of bursal sacs associated with muscles and tendons below the knee. Communication of the cyst with the knee joint may be demonstrated.

Clinical Findings. Swelling may be the only symptom noted, but in some patients the cyst may cause vague pain and discomfort associated with a sensation of giving-way of the knee.

Treatment. The cyst may be aspirated and injected with corticosteroids. Surgical excision may be required based on the intensity of the symptoms, or repeated aspiration and injection may be performed.

Trigger Thumb
Trigger thumb is the term used to describe momentary obstruction of the thumb when moved from the flexed to the extended position. Occasionally the thumb is locked in flexion.

Cause. It is caused by repeated trauma, which thickens the sheath of the flexor pollicis longus tendon.

Clinical Findings. A momentary lag is experienced when the thumb is brought from the flexed to the extended position. Occasionally the thumb is blocked in its flexed position and requires forceful extension. Pain may also be associated with gripping.

Treatment. Immobilization of the hand and thumb in a cast for several weeks will allow the swelling to subside. Other conservative measures include injection of local anesthetics and corticosteroids. Occasionally surgery is required; it consists of incision of the constricted area of the flexed tendon sheath.

Dupuytren's Contracture
Dupuytren's contracture is a contracture of the palmar aponeurosis that may produce a flexion deformity of the involved fingers. Its cause is unknown.

Clinical Findings. This condition is more frequently seen in males than in females. It usually begins with a nodule in the palm at the distal palmar crease proximal to the ring finger. This condition is chronic and may take anywhere from 1 to 20 years to reach its maximum deformity. The main complaint is one of deformity and interference with the use of the hand by the flexed fingers.

Treatment. Surgical release of the deforming scar tissue is performed.

Ganglion
Ganglion is the term used to describe a cystic swelling overlying a joint. It may be due to degeneration in the connective tissues close to the joint tendon sheaths; however, the exact etiology is unknown.

Clinical Findings. Ganglia occur about the wrist, most commonly on the dorsal surface. They may occur gradually or suddenly, and trauma may be a factor.

Treatment. Aspiration of the fluid contents and injection of corticosteroids is usually the treatment of choice and has a high rate of success. Surgical excision may be necessary in persistent cases when symptoms warrant.

Morton's Neuroma
Morton's neuroma is a swelling and neuromatous formation in an interdigital nerve of the foot.

Clinical Findings. The patient is frequently a middle-aged woman who complains of aching and burning in the foot, usually between the third and fourth metatarsals. The discomfort is relieved by removing the shoe and rubbing the foot.

Treatment. A metatarsal bar, loose footwear, or injection with local anesthetics and corticosteroids can be helpful. Surgical excision of the neuroma is curative and is indicated when conservative treatment fails (Fig. 3-47).

Scoliosis
Scoliosis is the term used to describe lateral deviation and rotation of a series of vertebrae from the midline anatomic po-

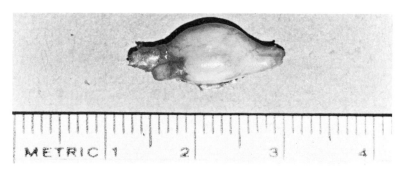

Figure 3-47. Excised Morton's neuroma.

sition of the normal spinal axis. The spine looks curved when viewed from the frontal plane.

Cause. Scoliosis may be due to functional or postural causes or may be secondary to affections of the neuromusculoskeletal system. Most commonly, scoliosis is idiopathic (no known origin).

Pathology. Abnormalities range from no fixed deformities, as in a functional scoliosis, to actual wedging of the vertebrae and fixed changes in the bony structures.

Clinical Findings. In functional scoliosis the curve is usually long, with little rotation, and the patient can voluntarily straighten the spine. In structural scoliosis, there is a fixed curvature of the spine and a rotational component, so that when the patient bends forward there is prominence of the posterior structures of the body on the convex side of the curve posteriorly and on the concave side of the curve anteriorly. In this most common type of right thoracic idiopathic scoliosis, when the patient bends forward the right rib cage is prominent posteriorly on the right and anteriorly on the left.

X-ray Findings. X-ray studies show that the functional scoliotic curve can be straightened without any bony deformity. The structural scoliotic curve is not correctable passively or actively and on x-rays there is wedging of the vertebral bodies with some rotary deformity.

Treatment. Functional scoliosis in itself does not require treatment. If it is secondary to a problem of the hip or the lower extremity, then correction of the extremity disorder will straighten the functional scoliosis. The treatment of structural scoliosis begins with correcting the underlying disorder if this is possible. The most common cause of scoliosis, however, is idiopathic, and in this case treatment is directed toward prevention of progression of the curvature, which most commonly occurs during the phase of rapid growth, and toward straightening the already significantly curved back. Treatment is complicated. Often traction for correction of the curvature and prolonged special bracing procedures are necessary. If conservative measures and bracing do not control the development of the scoliosis, then operative correction with the use of internal instrumentation and spinal fusion may be indicated.

OTHER SIGNIFICANT DISEASES
Diabetes
In the nursing care plan of orthopedic patients, one must keep in mind the fact that diabetes does cause peripheral neuritis and neuropathy as well as peripheral vasculitis in many cases. A clinical manifestation is decreased sensation, which subjects extremities to excessive trauma and poor cir-

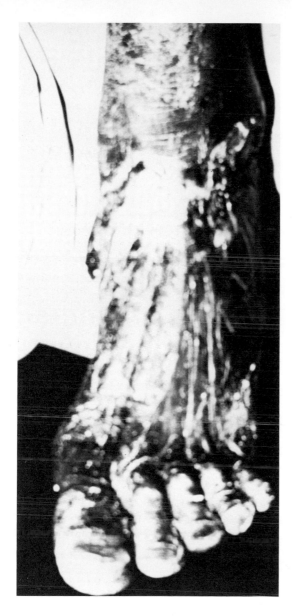

Figure 3-48, Gangrene of the left foot secondary to severe peripheral vascular disease.

culation, both factors conducive to acute and chronic infection. Treatment of diabetic problems is primarily directed toward prevention, meticulous hygiene, and avoidance of minor trauma. Once chronic infection and osteomyelitis occur in a diabetic they are very difficult to eradicate, and amputation may be necessary.

Cardiac Disease
Cardiac disease is especially significant in postinjury and postoperative orthopedic management. The use of a walker and

crutches requires considerable exertion, as does managing the extremity in a cast. One must take into consideration the overall status of the individual and adjust the physical activities to within his or her tolerance.

Peripheral Vascular Disease
Peripheral vascular disease is significant in the treatment of all orthopedic conditions in that diminished circulation to an extremity can predispose it to infection, slow healing, and skin pressure sores (Fig. 3-48).

Gastrointestinal Disease
Gastrointestinal disease can produce malabsorption syndromes with low calcium levels and adult osteomalacia.

SUGGESTED READINGS

Adams, J.C.: *Outline of Orthopedics* (7th ed.). Baltimore: Williams and Wilkins, 1971.

Baden, Ann Marie: Children with arthritis, some everyday help. *Nursing '73*, pp. 22–24, December 1973.

Dehaemers, Robert J., et al.: Rupture of the cervical disc. *Nursing '73*: 33–37, April 1973.

DiPalma, Joseph R.: Recent developments in bone-disease treatment. *R.N.* 36:63–72, January 1973.

Doswell, Willa M.: Sickle cell disease. *Nursing '74*, pp. 18–22, June 1974.

Ehtisham, M.: Osteoporosis. *Nurs. Times* 70:1544–1546, 1974.

Farrell, Jane: Wound infection and gas gangrene. *Orthop. Nurs. Assoc. J.* 2:64–65, March 1975.

Gartland, John J.: *Fundamentals of Orthopedics* (2nd ed.). Philadelphia: Saunders, 1974.

Golding, D.N.: Acute backache. *Nurs. Times* 70:184–185, 1974.

Gutman, Alexander B.: Views on the pathogenesis and management of primary gout — 1971. *J. Bone Joint Surg.* 54 [Am]:357–372, 1972.

Hastings, David E., and Hewitson, W.A.: Double hemiarthroplasty of the knee in rheumatoid arthritis. *J. Bone Joint Surg.* 55 [Br]:112–118, 1973.

Jacobs, Philip: Tumours of bone. *Nurs. Times* 68:1572–1575, 1972.

Millard, F.J.C.: Paget's disease. *Nurs. Times* 68:497–499, 1972.

Ryan, John: Compression in bone healing. *Am. J. Nurs.* 74:1998–1999, 1974.

Schumann, Delores, and Patterson, Phyllis: Multiple myeloma. *Am. J. Nurs.* 75:78–81, 1975.

Soika, Cynthia Vaughan: Combatting osteoporosis. *Am. J. Nurs.* 73:1193–1197, 1973.

Thomas, Betty J.: Recognizing and treating arthritis in the young. *R.N.* 37:64–68, September 1974.

Turek, S.L.: *Orthopaedics: Principles and Their Application* (2nd ed.). Philadelphia: Lippincott, 1967.

Warr, A.C.: Acute low back pain. *Nurs. Mirror* 137:47–49, September 1973.

Wells, Robert E.: Lumbar laminectomy and/or fusions. *Orthop. Nurs. Assoc. J.* 1:33–36, September 1974.

4. PLAN FOR NURSING CARE

The nursing care plan cannot be devised without a basic knowledge of those disease processes, conditions, or types of trauma which affect the neuromusculoskeletal system as well as of the current clinical management and surgical treatment of these processes or conditions.

According to *Standards of Orthopedic Nursing Practice,* as developed by the Orthopedic Nurses' Association, Inc., and the American Nurses' Association, Division of Medical-Surgical Nursing Practice, the nursing care plan "prescribes nursing actions to achieve the goals." Furthermore, the plan includes: "setting of priorities for appropriate nursing actions; a logical sequence of actions to attain the goals."*

The plan must incorporate specific nursing actions in regard to patient and family education, principles of fracture treatment (when applicable), the appropriate use of orthopedic devices, minimum compromise to related body systems, and anticipated complications. These nursing actions must be identified further as to how, when, where, and by whom they are to be accomplished.*

A well developed care plan is obviously useless unless it can be implemented effectively to provide optimum care to the patient. Furthermore, the care plan must be continuously updated following reassessment and reevaluation.

All persons involved in the care of the patient must be knowledgeable concerning the care plan as well as the rationale for the specific actions. To perform tasks rotely is to negate the plan of care. The patient and his or her family must be involved not only in the planning phases of care, but in the implementation phase as well.

GOALS

There are nursing goals as well as patient goals and both may be necessary in the plan of care. A nursing goal is a statement of intent of a nursing action(s); it is to be the end result of that action(s). Conversely, a patient goal is one in which the end result will be a change in the patient's behavior. He or she will know, have a change in attitude, or be able to demonstrate that which is changed from the original; nursing ac-

*From *Standards of Orthopedic Nursing Practice* as developed by the Orthopedic Nurses' Association, Inc., and the American Nurses' Association, Division of Medical-Surgical Nursing Practice, 1975.

tion(s) are also directed toward this goal. "The *goal* of *ortho-pedic nursing* is to restore and maintain maximum function of the neuromusculoskeletal system."*

Goals should be written in terms of patient outcomes. There are known patient outcomes specific to individuals requiring orthopedic nursing care. These patient outcomes are: "the individual or responsible party demonstrates a knowledge of his disorder and how this may permanently or temporarily modify his life"; "the individual or responsible party utilizes modalities of orthopedic treatment for maximum benefit"; "the individual or responsible party demonstrates the appropriate responses to orthopedic intervention"; "the individual or responsible party realizes that he [the individual] is the primary rehabilitative resource"; "the individual or responsible party is free from preventable adverse effects from modalities of orthopedic treatment and nursing action."*

Goals are established following the nursing and medical diagnosis. They must be realistic and thus attainable within an established period of time. Furthermore, they must be assigned an order of preference based on urgency or relative importance. To set goals in any other manner is not only unfair to the patient, but also frustrating to the personnel involved in his or her care.

THE CARE PLAN

The format of nursing care plans varies from institution to institution; however, all plans should include the nursing diagnosis, medical diagnosis, goals, and specific nursing actions. The rationale for each specific action should also be included. The following information will enable the reader to develop specific care plans from a broad base of orthopedic nursing principles of patient care.

General Care

TURNING THE ORTHOPEDIC PATIENT. The following principles apply to the turning of most orthopedic patients with back, hip, or lower extremity problems. The steps that incorporate these principles make the turning procedure possible with minimal discomfort to the patient and without complicating the basic orthopedic or postoperative problem. Except in unusual instances, as ordered by the physician, the patient is turned away from the involved extremity.

It is vital to explain to the patient that turning will be done

*From *Standards of Orthopedic Nursing Practice* as developed by the Orthopedic Nurses' Association, Inc., and the American Nurses' Association, Division of Medical-Surgical Nursing Practice, 1975.

carefully, and that nothing will be done to compromise the surgical results or intensify the injury. Reassuring the patient in this manner will reduce muscle spasm and tension and is often worth more than a narcotic.

If the patient is able to help in turning, depending on the physician's instructions, the side rail toward which the patient will be turned is pulled up. Instruct the patient to reach across and firmly grasp this side rail as he is being turned so that he can help the nurse to turn him on his side. Also explain that as he is being turned an assistant will gently and carefully support the leg that has been injured or operated on and place it on two pillows so that undue stress will not be placed on it. The patient should always be told about this assistance before the actual turning maneuvers begin. It is also advisable to tell the patient that the physician has left instructions for him to be turned, and that even though turning may cause some discomfort, the overall result will be increased comfort and minimization of convalescent care problems.

After giving the patient preliminary instructions and reassurance, obtain enough help and pillows to support the legs.

With pillows positioned in the bed so that they are readily available, stand on the side toward which the patient will be turned. Reach across the patient's chest and trunk, placing your upper hand behind the far shoulder and your lower hand behind the far side of the pelvis. (The lower hand is on the crest of the pelvis and not directly over the hip joint.)

A second person will be needed to help at this point if the patient has had a hip operation or has an injured leg in a long cast. This assistant gently supports the involved extremity, after removing it from traction when this is necessary.

Gently turn the patient on one side. Pillows are used for support in this position, thus freeing the assistant to help with the leg. Carefully position two or three pillows under the involved extremity, allowing it to flex slightly for comfort while maintaining it in a slightly abducted position; that is, out to the side at all times. This position is safe for almost any patient who has had hip surgery. It is most important not to let the affected extremity drop down in front of the body into adduction. The adducted position could damage a hip nailing and cause a prosthesis or arthroplasty to dislocate. With the patient turned on the uninvolved side and the pillows adjusted under the injured extremity, adjust the head pillow and place more pillows or folded blankets behind the patient's back and tuck them under to keep him from rolling.

Turning the patient in bed is beneficial for several reasons, including the following: there is less likelihood of complications such as respiratory infection, urinary infection, or thrombophlebitis, because turning and repositioning a patient promotes circulation and respiratory excursion, and prevents urinary stasis. Also, back care is facilitated, pressure areas can be prevented, and the patient is made more comfortable, as turning relieves muscle spasm and tension produced by lying in one position for a long period of time.

USE OF THE OVERHEAD TRAPEZE. The overhead trapeze is probably the single most important tool in the nursing care of the orthopedic patient. It is primarily used for patient comfort and back care. The use of an overhead trapeze is predicated on the patient's ability to use the upper extremities. The trapeze enables the patient to move about or be transferred or lifted for use of the bedpan and back care, the normal upper extremities substituting for the muscles of the trunk and involved extremities.

Usually the overhead trapeze is adjusted so that the patient can comfortably lift himself up and grasp it with both hands, with the elbows in a position of approximately 30 degrees of flexion. From this position the patient can further flex the elbows comfortably, gaining the additional distance necessary to lift the back and pelvis off the bed.

Advantageous use of the overhead trapeze, however, depends on educating the patient in its correct use. If an overhead trapeze is simply hung on the bed and the patient is told to use it, he will use it, but may well do himself harm, particularly if he has preexisting back problems. The patient must be instructed in how to lift his back, buttocks, and shoulders off the bed in a straight line; otherwise he will often grab the trapeze, raise his head and shoulders up, and force his pelvis against the bed. This position is contraindicated in patients with back difficulties and obviously would not facilitate skin care and use of the bedpan. The overhead trapeze is also used by the patient and nursing personnel in transferring from bed to stretcher or chair.

PELVIC LIFT. For a patient to be able to use a bedpan with a minimum amount of effort and discomfort, it is important that he be given a careful explanation of how to do this. With care, specific instructions, and help, a patient with a hip in traction or with a long leg cast or recent back surgery, can successfully use a bedpan without undue discomfort or damage. The minimum requirements are that the patient have functional upper extremities, one strong, functional uninvolved lower extremity, and an overhead trapeze. The steps in teaching a patient to maneuver a pelvic lift are as follows:

Explain to the patient what you are going to teach him to do. Assure him that he will be able to do it without injuring himself. Caution him to give you time for a complete explanation, as often when you first tell a patient that you are going to teach him how to get on a bedpan he reaches up, grasps the trapeze, and starts pulling the head and shoulders up toward the trapeze, forcing the buttocks against the bed. That is, he will do exactly what he should not be doing in order to use the bedpan properly.

Have the patient place his hands on the overhead trapeze. Instruct him that when he pulls and lifts himself up he is not to raise his head and shoulders up toward the trapeze, but is to keep them straight and level with the buttocks so that the entire body will rise off the bed as a unit (Fig. 4-1).

Instruct and assist the patient in bending the uninjured lower extremity (or both extremities if neither extremity is injured or incapacitated) at the knee and placing the foot (or feet) as flat as possible on the bed (Fig. 4-2).

With his hands positioned on the overhead trapeze and the uninvolved lower extremity in the correct position, instruct the patient to push down with the foot that is flat on the bed

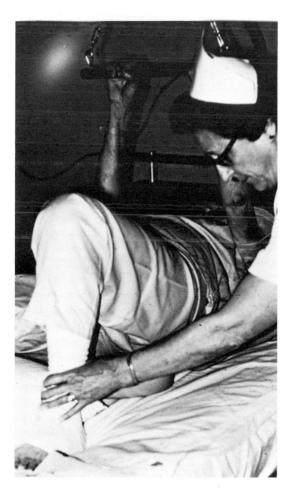

Figure 4-1. Pelvic lift.

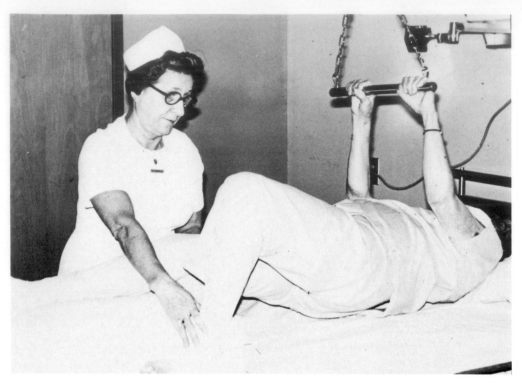

Figure 4-2. Pelvic lift for a patient unable to use one lower extremity.

(often a stabilizing hand on the foot will keep the patient from slipping) and at the same time to pull on the trapeze, allowing the entire body and trunk to rise off the bed. Again, stress that the head and shoulders are not to be raised higher than the buttocks, but that the shoulders, back, and buttocks are to move as a straight unit.

As the patient's trunk and buttocks rise off the bed, the bedpan may be placed in the proper position, back care given, or the bed made. (Often a fracture bedpan will be easier for the patient to use than a conventional bedpan, as it does not require the patient to lift himself high off the surface of the bed.)

If a patient is in a weakened condition, one or two assistants may be necessary to enable the patient to perform this procedure. One assistant can place a hand under the shoulders or sacral area so that not as much strength is required to lift the body off the bed. If both lower extremities are involved, assistants can substitute for the legs by supporting the patient with a hand under the sacrum and shoulders (Fig. 4-3).

Always remember to explain carefully to the patient what you wish him to do.

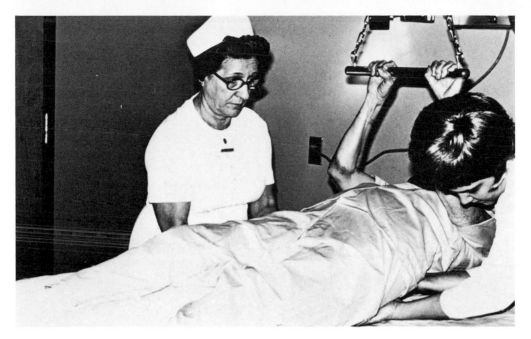

Figure 4-3. Pelvic lift for patient unable to use either lower extremity.

USE OF AN EXERCISE SLING. A simple exercise sling may be used to assist a patient with hip and knee motion as well as to facilitate movement of an extremity which has been injured or operated on.

To set up an exercise sling, the following materials are needed in addition to a full length overhead frame: a knee sling, a spreader bar, a rope, and a handle. The rope is attached to a spreader bar and run through a pulley on a side bar above the patient's knee and through another pulley on a side bar above the patient's arm. The knee sling is then positioned under the knee and attached to a spreader bar (Fig. 4-4).

The patient can then pull on the handle and give himself gentle, assisted hip and knee flexion (Fig. 4-5). If the sling is positioned under the calf of the involved leg, the patient can pull on the handle and lift the leg off the bed, giving himself active, assisted hip abduction and adduction as well as knee extension (Fig. 4-6). The sling can also be used as an assistive device for movement of the extremity when changing positions.

The knee sling is a simple way to allow the patient to contribute to his own rehabilitation.

NEUROVASCULAR CHECKS OF AN EXTREMITY. Careful evaluation must be made of the extremity following injury, surgery, or any condition requiring casting or traction. The

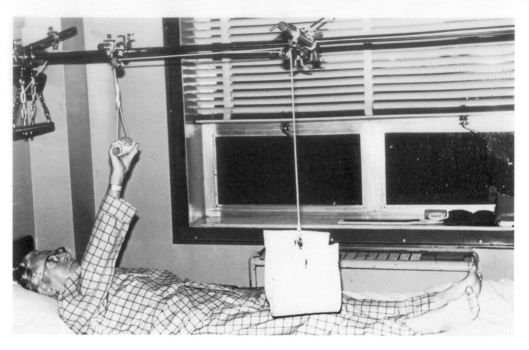

Figure 4-4. Exer-
cise sling for the
right leg.

Figure 4-5. Active
assisted range of
motion of the
right knee and hip
with an exercise
sling.

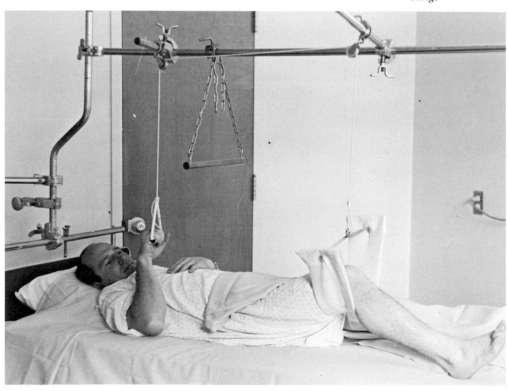

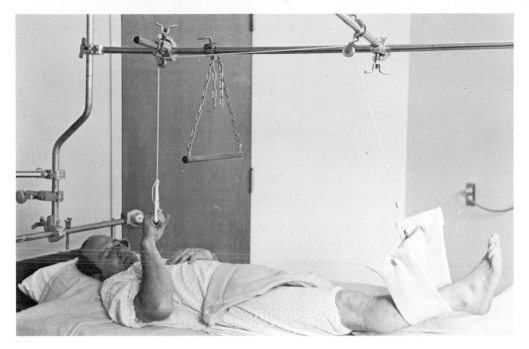

Figure 4-6. Knee extension and hip motion with an exercise sling.

extremity must be observed and notes recorded accurately. The frequency of the checks depends on the injury and the precariousness of the situation. In general, neurovascular checks are done every 1 to 2 hours for the first 24 hours and are continued if there is any risk in discontinuing them.

Swelling. The swelling of the distal extremity must be evaluated and can be described as mild, moderate, or severe. Swelling can cause grave complications because it may occlude arterial supply and venous return, resulting in tissue ischemia and necrosis.

Color. The color of the distal extremity is evaluated in comparison with the opposite extremity, and is usually described as normal, bluish, or pale. A bluish color is indicative of obstructed venous return, whereas pallor usually means that there is decreased arterial supply.

Temperature. The temperature of the distal extremity is also evaluated in comparison with the opposite extremity and can be recorded as normal, cold, or hot. A decreased blood supply may be indicated if the extremity is cool or cold. If the extremity is too warm there may be decreased venous return or an infection. However, one must always consider that the coolness may be simply due to ice bags around the extremity or an air conditioner blowing directly on the extremity. This check must be viewed in conjunction with other neurovascular checks.

Pulses. Pulses of the involved extremity are evaluated and described as strong, weak, or absent. Often pulses cannot be checked due to the cast or dressing.

Capillary Filling. Capillary filling is evaluated by compressing the distal finger or toe (or nail) firmly and comparing the rate at which it attains its normal color with this rate on the uninvolved side. Capillary filling is described as normal, sluggish, or absent. A sluggish return or no return of color is usually due to a decreased arterial supply, which may be secondary to vessel trauma, pressure, or arterial occlusion.

Motion. Motion of the extremity distal to the injury or surgery must be properly evaluated. Having the patient wiggle his fingers or toes is *not* a proper evaluation. The patient must be asked to actually flex or extend the fingers or toes, first actively and then passively. If there is a mechanical restriction, such as a pin in a finger or toe, which would prevent flexion or extension, obviously this should not be attempted. However, if there is no mechanical restriction of motion, any lack of motion should be reported to the physician. Pain with passive motion should be reported immediately.

Sensation. The patient's description of sensation in response to application of heat and cold and to light, sharp, and dull touch should be recorded. Any tingling sensation must also be noted. Decreasing sensation may be caused by actual nerve damage, pressure on the nerve, or decreased blood supply. Progressive loss of sensation must be reported immediately.

Pain. Progressive, unrelieved pain is the most valid indicator of impending vascular compromise. It is usually the first change noted in the extremity and must be reported immediately. These patients clinically appear anxious, restless, and generally uncomfortable and continue to complain of pain even after given medication that would normally control postoperative discomfort. A patient with these symptoms must have a complete neurovascular check done immediately and the surgeon must be notified. This is an orthopedic emergency.

PAIN. Although the bone has no nerve supply, the periosteum surrounding it is quite sensitive; therefore, postoperatively or posttraumatically orthopedic patients usually experience severe pain. One should remember that in a fracture or a surgical procedure the soft tissues surrounding the bone have also been injured, resulting in contractile activity that produces pain. Appropriate nursing measures such as elevation, support, and positioning of the affected part should be performed, as well as the administration of analgesics and narcotics as ordered.

Nursing Care of the Patient in Traction
Traction is frequently considered a rope and pulley monster. The patient in traction must be viewed with a basic understanding of the reasons for this type of treatment.

The pulling force applied to an extremity or other part of the body, either manually or by mechanical means, is called *traction*. There are many different types of traction, but most of them fall into one of three general categories: skin traction, which is applied to the skin and soft tissues (the pull is applied indirectly to the skeletal system) (Fig. 4-7); skeletal traction, which is applied directly to the skeletal system by a Steinmann pin, Kirschner wire, Crutchfield tongs, or other device (Fig. 4-8); and manual traction, which is a pulling force applied to a part of the body by the hands. These definitions are not given to be memorized, but to assist in recognizing the patient's type of traction.

There are many reasons for the patient to be in traction. Traction is used to immobilize an extremity and thereby allow it to rest; to correct or prevent flexion deformities of the knee or hip of the patient with arthritis; to relieve or reduce muscle spasm in the patient with a fractured hip, back pain, or other condition; and to maintain the alignment of a fracture that has been reduced.

After determining the type of traction the patient is in and why it is being used, stand by the bed and look at the traction

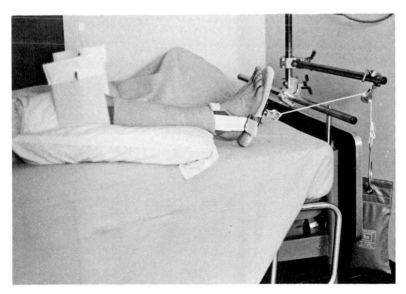

Figure 4-7. Skin traction for the right leg.

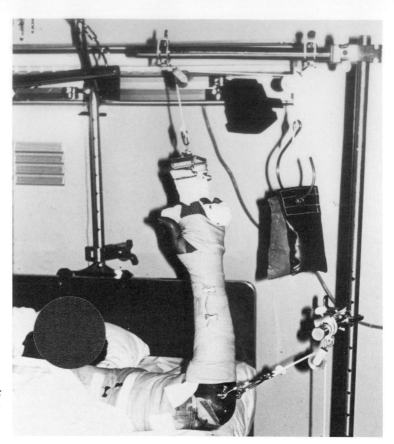

Figure 4-8. Skeletal traction utilizing a pin through the left olecranon; the forearm is suspended by skin traction.

setup. Realize that every rope is attached to something. Follow the rope from where it is attached, noting that it will go over a pulley (occasionally more than one) and attach to a weight. Often there will be several ropes, pulleys, and weights, but after determining where they all come from or attach to and where they lead, it becomes clear that the rope and pulley monster is a logical assembly.

Alignment and countertraction are two terms frequently used in association with traction, and it is important that they be understood before one attempts to care for a patient. *Alignment* simply means keeping the part of the body in traction in line with the pull of the weight. *Countertraction* is a force exerted in the direction opposite to the pull produced by the traction; it balances the applied traction. The countertraction is usually the patient's own body weight. For example, if traction has been applied to the lower extremities, the patient is instructed to keep himself pulled up toward the head of the bed to maintain countertraction. If the patient is a child or a thin adult (light body weight), the foot of the bed may have to be elevated to maintain traction and prevent the patient from being pulled down in the bed by the traction.

Traction is never released unless this is ordered by the physician. Never remove a weight, lay a weight on the bed, or lower it to the floor unless you have an order. By the same token, straps or wrappings are not removed without direct instructions. There are many types of traction that may be released for a period of time or in which straps may be rewrapped, but there must always be an order for this. This is a decision the nurse does not make in the care of the patient in traction. If the physician writes an order to release the traction or rewrap the straps, he does so knowing that if the nurse handles the involved part carefully, there will be no injurious effects to the patient.

Even in traction, the patient has more liberty of movement than one would think possible. Most nursing procedures can be carried out without hurting the patient or disrupting the traction. A bath, linen change, back care, and the elimination of body wastes can and should be accomplished efficiently. The physician expects these activities to be carried out for the patient. Use of the bedpan and back care can both be accomplished by employing pelvic lift.

The bath is begun in the same manner as for any other patient. The upper back may be bathed by having the patient grasp the trapeze and lift his shoulders off the bed. The lower back, sacral area, and buttocks may be bathed and back care given by following the simple pelvic lift procedure.

The linen change is accomplished in the following manner: Clean linen is placed on the side of the bed, under the patient's uninvolved limb. Then, with an assistant on the opposite side of the bed, the patient's hips and shoulders are lifted, employing pelvic lift. The clean linen is spread under the patient, the soiled linen having been pushed to the opposite side. The soiled linen is removed and the bedmaking finished. In some cases it may be easier to make the bed from top to bottom or bottom to top instead of from side to side. Most patients in traction will not be allowed to turn from side to side.

In caring for a patient in traction, it is important to be flexible with all nursing procedures. The most important tool that the nurse and patient have for achieving some mobility is the overhead trapeze.

Certain important considerations and precautions apply to all patients in traction. These considerations are: assisting the patient in pulling himself up in bed at frequent intervals during the day; realizing that traction will not be accomplished if the footplate or the knot in the rope is in contact with the pulley or the foot of the bed; and being aware of the fact that friction caused by ropes riding on the foot of the bed, ropes

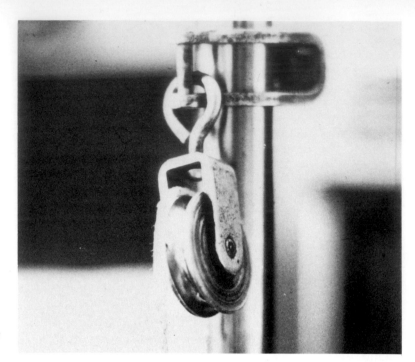

Figure 4-9. Rope off pulley.

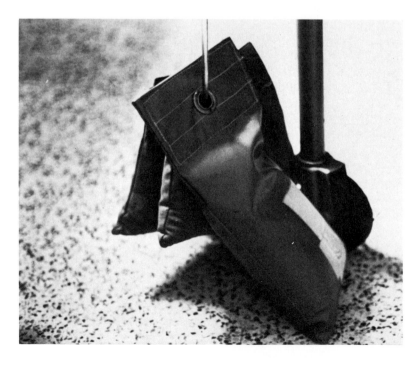

Figure 4-10. Weights on floor.

caught in the bedclothes or off the pulley (Fig. 4-9), or heels digging into the mattress lessen the efficiency of the traction. Also, be sure that weights do not touch the floor (Fig. 4-10), drag on bed parts, or catch against other weight systems. All weights must hang free, and only on orders from the physician is traction weight added or removed. Skin sores due to the pressure from the traction apparatus or body weight in areas of poor natural padding must be avoided. Danger points that are subject to pressure or body weight include the bony prominences about the elbow, the wrist, the ankle, the hip, the bony prominence at the neck of the fibula, the backs of the heels, and the prominences of the sacrum, spine, scapulas, and pelvis (Figs. 4-11, 4-12). Make certain that body alignment and the position of the extremity are maintained; make frequent checks of the circulation and sensation of the extremity in traction; and encourage coughing, deep breathing, and any activity the patient can comfortably do in traction.

The patient who is to be in continuous traction postoperatively or posttraumatically needs a tremendous amount of emotional support from all those dealing with him. Although many patients will never voice their fears, they find the traction apparatus overwhelming.

Boredom is a very real problem and unless diversional activities are offered, the patient may become depressed.

Although these guidelines do not tell how to give specific care to a given patient, the principles are basic. When caring for a patient in traction, first read the chart and find out the reason for the traction. Then, take time to find out where the traction ropes attach to the patient, and therefore what their pull will tend to do. You can confidently and efficiently care for the patient by understanding the purpose of the traction and the basic principles involved.

MANUAL TRACTION. Manual traction is used in the aligning of fractures prior to casting or to hold an extremity until traction can be applied.

BUCK'S TRACTION. Buck's traction is a type of skin traction most frequently used in the care of hip fractures or when there is a joint irritation of the hip or knee (Fig. 4-13). Usually the maintenance of this traction is not critical and it may be removed temporarily for skin care when so ordered by the physician.

SPLIT RUSSELL'S TRACTION. Split Russell's traction is Buck's traction with an additional weighted knee sling (Fig. 4-14). It is used frequently after arthroplasty of the hip, in the treatment of fractures of the femur, and for injured or diseased hips and knees. The physician often allows its removal for skin care if its maintenance is not critical.

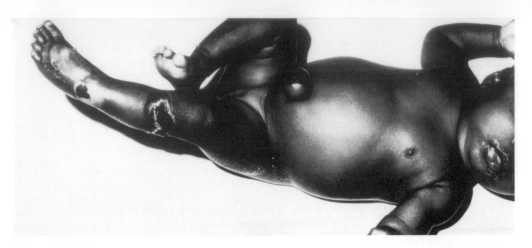

Figure 4-11. Contracture of the left leg secondary to improperly applied and maintained Bryant's traction.

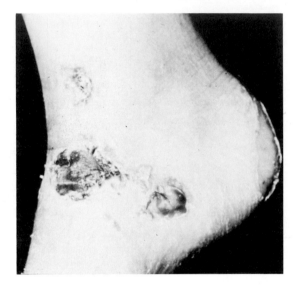

Figure 4-12. Pressure areas on the foot and ankle secondary to improperly applied and padded traction.

Figure 4-13. Buck's traction for the right leg.

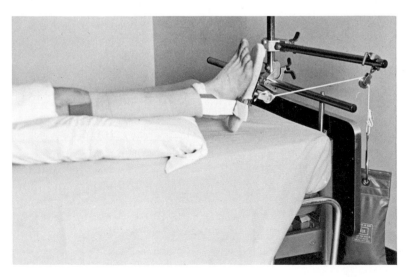

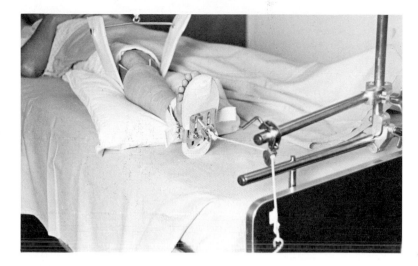

Figure 4-14. Split Russell's traction for the right leg.

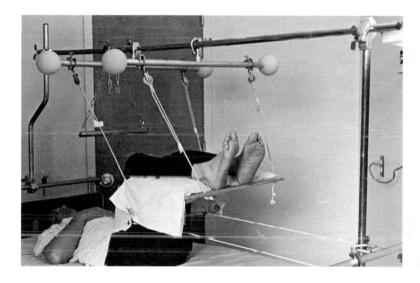

Figure 4-15. 90–90 pelvic traction.

90–90 PELVIC TRACTION. This form of traction is usually used in the conservative management of patients with back pain. The hips and knees are placed in 90 degrees of flexion and traction is applied to the thighs (Fig. 4-15). The schedule for this varies according to the physician's orders. Some patients are unable to tolerate this traction for long periods of time.

PELVIC TRACTION. Pelvic traction is also a type of skin traction utilized to relieve muscle spasm in the patient with low back pain. Traction is applied over the pelvic girdle (Fig. 4-16).

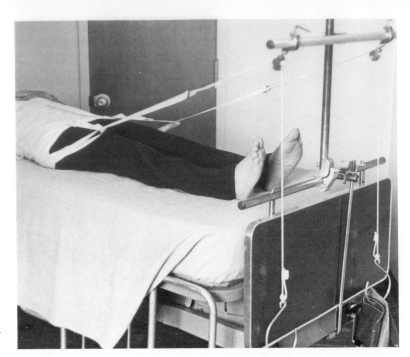

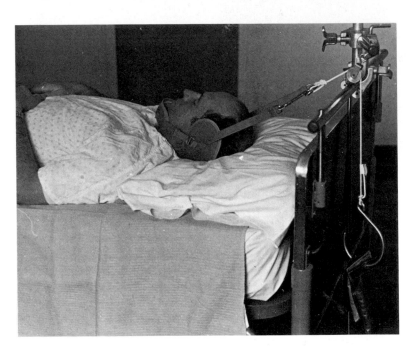

Figure 4-16. Pelvic traction.

Figure 4-17. Cervical traction.

CERVICAL TRACTION. This is a form of skin traction used to relieve muscle spasm and pain caused by cervical disc disease or a muscle injury (Fig. 4-17). The position of the head may vary for the patient's comfort or with the physician's preference. Skin cervical traction must be released intermittently

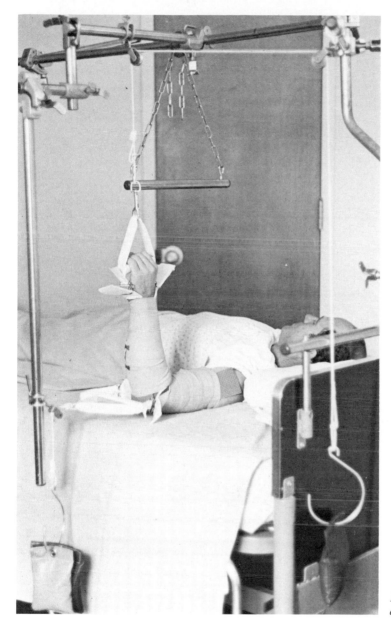

Figure 4-18. Side arm traction.

and the areas of pressure rubbed with the fingers, to avoid pressure sores. Cervical traction cannot be tolerated 24 hours a day without skin breakdown. If constant cervical traction is required, skeletal traction will be used.

SIDE ARM TRACTION. This type of skin traction may be used postoperatively or after injury to maintain proper anatomic position (Fig. 4-18). Neurovascular checks must be performed routinely. If weights pull the patient toward the

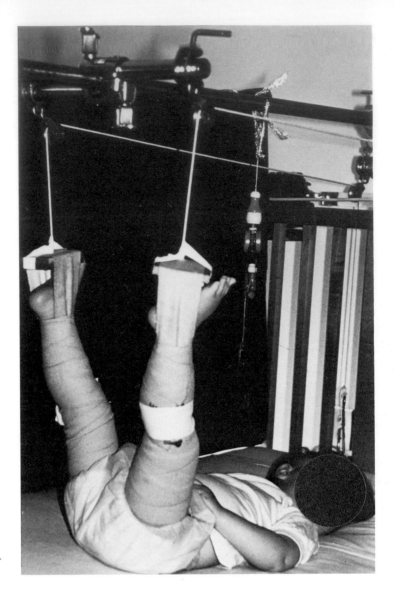

Figure 4-19. Bry-ant's traction.

traction, place blocks under the bed on the affected side or put a rolled blanket between the mattress and the springs to tilt the patient away from the traction. Make sure a hand support is incorporated into the traction to maintain hand position and encourage finger and wrist motion. Although this type of traction usualiy cannot be released, inspect the skin underneath the wrapping routinely.

BRYANT'S TRACTION. Bryant's traction is used in the treatment of a fractured femur. Traction is applied through the skin of the lower extremity and the leg is suspended with the hip flexed at 90 degrees and the knee in full extension (Fig. 4-19). It is used only in children who weigh less than 30 to 35 pounds.

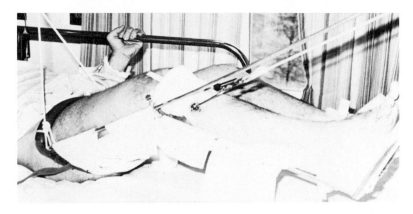

Figure 4-20. Balanced suspension with skeletal traction for the tibia.

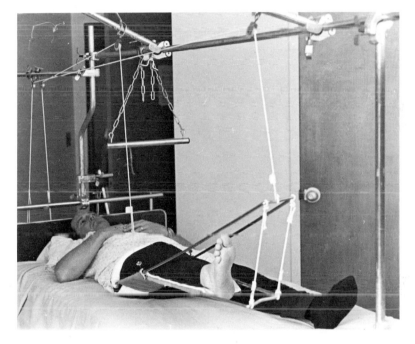

Figure 4-21. Balanced suspension.

BALANCED SUSPENSION. Balanced suspension is utilized in the treatment of the lower extremity after injury or surgery, when it is desirable for the entire leg to be supported free of the bed. If traction is also desired it may be combined with the balanced suspension by means of skeletal or skin traction (Figs. 4-20, 4-21). The extremity is placed in a covered splint (usually a Thomas variety), most commonly with a Pearson attachment to support the lower leg. The entire apparatus is then connected to a balancing system of ropes, pulleys, and weights. This allows the extremity to move comfortably up and down as the patient lifts his trunk off the bed.

COTREL'S TRACTION. Cotrel's traction is a combination of cervical and pelvic traction that is used to decrease spinal deformity. Weights are increased on a daily basis as ordered. Comfort measures include placing a small pillow under the legs and a small rolled towel under the neck; changing the position of the head halter; applying moist heat to the strained neck muscles, if allowed; and encouraging as much activity as possible within the limits of traction. Potential pressure areas are the occiput, heels, sacrum, iliac crest, ears, and chin. All these sites must be checked frequently.

HALO-FEMORAL TRACTION. This is a form of skeletal traction also used to decrease spinal deformities. Weights are increased on a daily basis. The pin sites in the skull and femurs must be checked frequently. Frequently assess potential pressure areas such as the heels and sacrum, as well as other bony prominences. Be alert for any neurologic warning signs such as numbness or tingling or complaints of visual disturbances. Encourage maximum activity within the limits of traction.

SKELETAL CERVICAL TRACTION. In this case, cervical traction is applied by way of Crutchfield, Barton, or Vinke tongs placed in the skull. This traction must be continuous. This form of traction is used in conjunction with a Stryker frame or Circolectric bed. The head-neck alignment must be maintained at all times in a neutral position. Should the tongs pull out, place a soft collar around the neck or immobilize the patient's head with sandbags and notify the physician immediately. Constant assessment of sensation and motion must be performed. Changes in sensation and loss of function are indicative of cord damage and the physician should be notified immediately. Check all potential pressure areas frequently; this should be done each time the patient is turned.

PIN CARE IN SKELETAL TRACTION. A sterile gauze dressing should be placed over the pin down to the pin site and left alone unless other orders are given (Fig. 4-22). A cork or adhesive tape is usually applied over the sharp ends of the wire or pin to protect the patient and personnel from injury.

TRACTION MATERIALS. Unless an over-the-head or over-the-foot type of traction device is to be used, such as cervical or Buck's traction, the bed must have an overhead frame applied before any form of traction may be set up. Assorted side bars, pulleys, 1/8-inch rope, and weights are needed to set up specific types of traction, as well as special materials such as a board for 90–90 traction, tongs for cervical skeletal traction, or a Thomas splint with a Pearson attachment for balanced suspension. The placement of the side bars and pulleys and the amount of weight used will depend on the purpose of the traction and the extremity to which it is being applied. Traction equipment varies with each institution, and one should

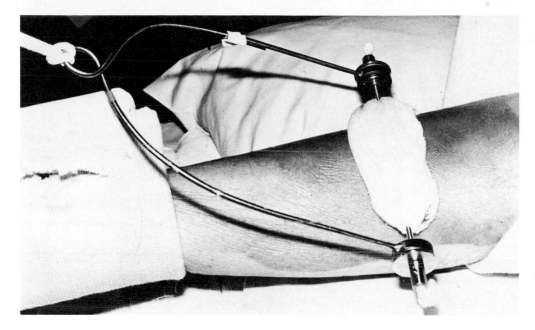

Figure 4-22. One type of skeletal pin traction dressing.

refer to the equipment book and procedures for the particular equipment at hand. Weights should be hung only at the foot and head of the bed as the patient may be unduly apprehensive if a weight is hanging over him.

Nursing Care of the Patient in a Cast

CAST APPLICATION. Casts are used for immobilization of the extremity postoperatively or posttraumatically. They are molded to the extremity and cover a large enough area to effectively immobilize the injured part (Figs. 4-23, 4-24, 4-25).

Plaster of Paris impregnated in a fabric base is most commonly utilized in preparation of casts. The reaction of plaster of Paris with water is exothermic and the heat of reaction can be felt by the patient on whom the cast is applied. Patients should be advised that this will occur so as to eliminate unnecessary concern. While a cast is setting, it should be exposed to the air and no plastic or rubber materials should be adjacent to or surrounding it, since excessive heating may occur, with burning of the patient's skin.

The *setting time* is the interval required for the material to become a rigid dressing. So-called green casts are those which have set, but from which the excess water has not evaporated; this takes from 24 to 72 hours, depending on the size of the cast.

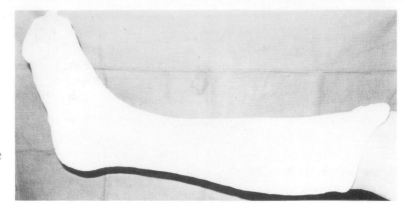

Figure 4-23. Short leg cast, patellar tendon bearing (PTB) type.

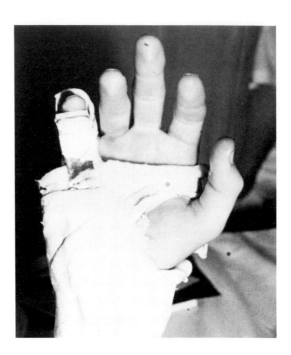

Figure 4-24. Short arm cast with splint for injured finger.

Materials necessary for the application of a cast are: padding such as stockinette and a soft cotton wrap; plaster rolls or splints; a bucket of warm water (operators vary in their preference of water temperature); any special materials required for a particular cast; and a cast saw, cast knife, and bandage scissors. The sizes and types of plaster and padding are determined by the part to be immobilized and the preference of the individual applying the cast.

Although it is a routine procedure for the personnel involved, having a cast applied is an undesirable and frightening experience for most patients. Therefore, a careful and com-

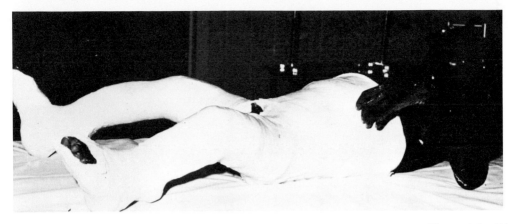

Figure 4-25. Bilateral long leg body-spica cast.

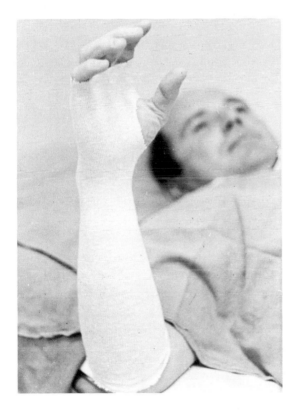

Figure 4-26. Stockinette placed on the extremity prior to casting.

plete explanation of the procedure must be given to the patient prior to the application of the cast.

The stockinette is placed on the involved extremity with great care being taken to allow no wrinkles (Fig. 4-26); this requires cutting the stockinette at the ankle joint or the elbow joint (Figs. 4-27, 4-28). The soft cotton padding is then ap-

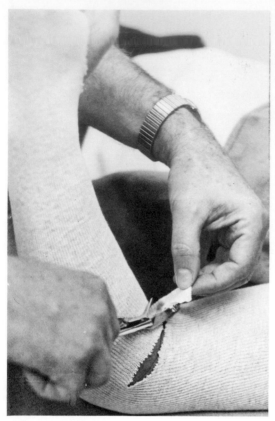

Figure 4-27. Excess stockinette is removed at the elbow crease.

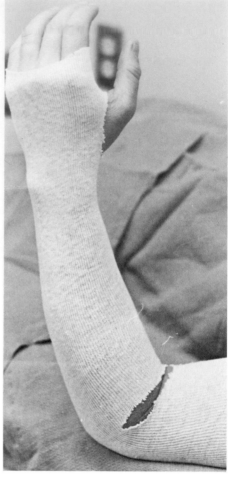

Figure 4-28. Cut stockinette prevents pressure at the elbow joint.

plied on top of the stockinette, overlapping approximately one-half thickness as the extremity is being covered (Figs. 4-29, 4-30). At the distal and proximal ends of the cast a couple of extra turns are applied to pad the edge of a cast, or a strip of felt may be used instead of extra rolls. An extra layer is also placed over the bony prominences such as the ulnar styloid process, malleoli, olecranon, and epicondyles. In fresh fractures the soft cotton wrapping only may be used.

When assisting with application of plaster, never dip the plaster until the operator is ready to apply it. The bandage is then removed from the paper wrapping and placed in the

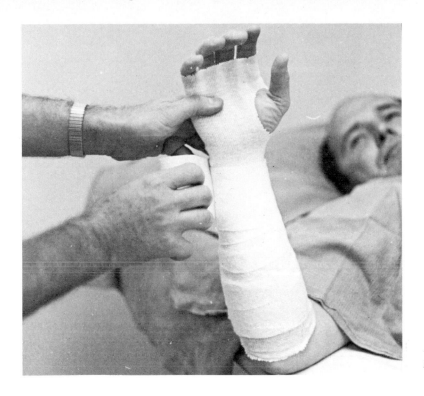

Figure 4-29. Ap-
plication of soft
cotton padding.

Figure 4-30.
Stockinette and
soft cotton pad-
ding in place.

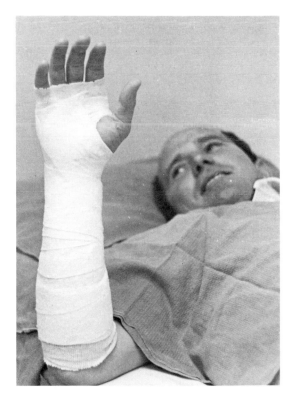

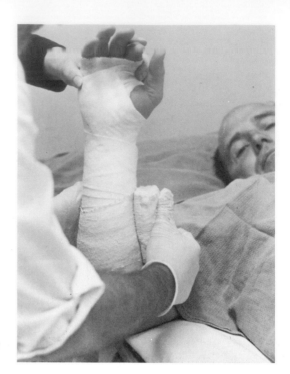

Figure 4-31. Plaster is rolled on the arm.

Figure 4-32. Tucks are taken in the plaster.

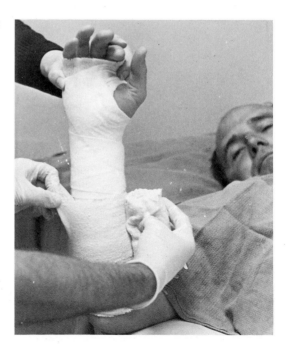

water with the end hanging free; the plaster is ready for application when the bubbling has stopped. The excess water is allowed to drain from the bandage when removing it from the water. Most operators prefer to have the excess water squeezed from the bandage; this is accomplished by holding the bandage roll with a hand at either end, crimping the edges, and giving it a gentle twist in opposite directions while gently squeezing with the fingers toward the middle. The plaster is then handed to the operator with the end out and hanging free.

The part to be immobilized must be placed in the required position before application of plaster. This position is maintained by an assistant during the application of plaster.

When applying plaster, push it around the part without lifting it off the surface, taking tucks in it as you move up and down (Figs. 4-31, 4-32). Never apply plaster under tension. As one hand is gently rolling the plaster on the extremity, the other hand rubs the already applied plaster, so that the end result is one layer rather than several layers, increasing the strength of the cast. Molding is accomplished with the palm of the hand and must be carried out until the plaster is set.

Short Arm Cast. Short arm casts should end below the bend of the elbow to allow elbow flexion (Fig. 4-33), and proximal to the distal palmar crease to allow metacarpophalangeal joint flexion (Figs. 4-34, 4-35). Usually only one layer of plaster goes between the thumb and index finger as this is the area where the bulk of the cast most commonly will rub and bother the patient (Fig. 4-36). Additional turns back and forth are made at the wrist area, as this is where most of the stress will be.

Long Arm Cast. Application of a long arm cast is essentially the same as that of a short arm cast. The elbow is immobilized at a 90-degree position which allows comfort and control of rotation (Fig. 4-37). Plaster is lapped back and forth behind the elbow joint, as this is the area that needs maximum support (Fig. 4-38).

Short Leg Cast. When a short leg cast is applied, it is important to hold the foot and ankle in the desired position rather than positioning them immediately after application, which will cause creasing, crinkling, and ridges in the cast (Fig. 4-39, 4-40). It is applied from just below the knee to the toes. Additional plaster is needed underneath the sole of the foot and around the ankle joint; this is accomplished by lapping the plaster roll back and forth underneath the sole of the foot and around the ankle rather than by rolling it around the foot and ankle. If a walking heel is to be applied this is done when the cast first becomes firm but is still damp. The walking heel is placed on the sole of the foot in the position of an imaginary

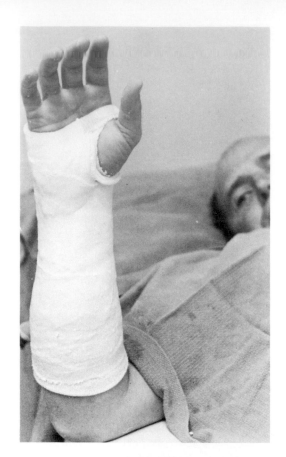

Figure 4-33. Completed short arm cast which allows elbow flexion.

Figure 4-34. The cast is trimmed proximal to the metacarpophalangeal joint.

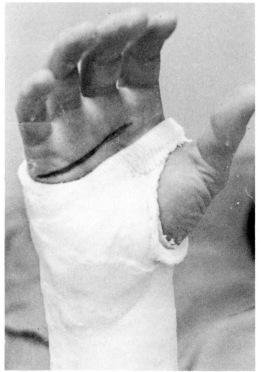

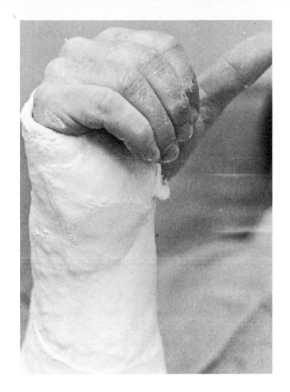

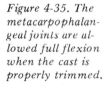
Figure 4-35. The metacarpophalangeal joints are allowed full flexion when the cast is properly trimmed.

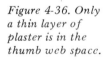
Figure 4-36. Only a thin layer of plaster is in the thumb web space.

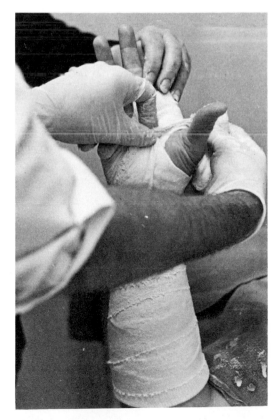

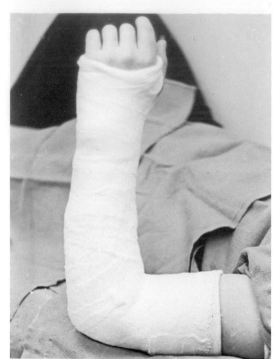

Figure 4-37. Completed long arm cast.

Figure 4-38. Reinforcing a long arm cast in an area of stress.

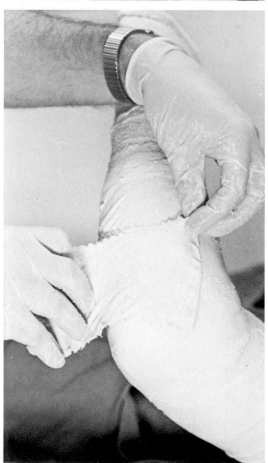

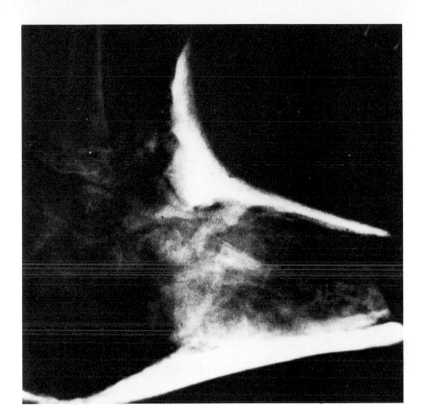

Figure 4-39. Excess plaster on the anterior aspect of the ankle due to positioning of the foot after plaster was first applied.

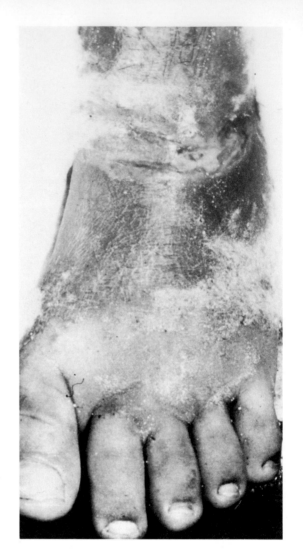

*Figure 4-40.
Necrosis of the
anterior aspect of
the ankle second-
ary to improper
application of
cast.*

line down the front of the tibia which would bisect the heel,
and is wrapped in place with a 3- or 4-inch roll of plaster. If a
commercial walking cast shoe is to be used, the sole of the cast
is made flat to afford a fit into the cast shoe. The cast over the
dorsum of the toes is usually cut away when the cast is becoming firm so that their neurovascular status can be evaluated and the toes can be exercised (Fig. 4-41). If weight bearing in the cast is to be allowed, the patient is instructed not
to begin this for 48 to 72 hours, since the cast continues to
dry and cure with increasing strength for this length of time.

Long Leg Cast. The long leg cast is applied as is the short
leg cast but it extends to the upper thigh (Fig. 4-42). The

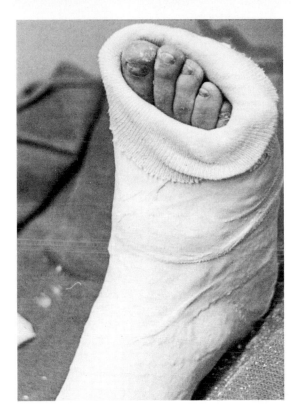

Figure 4-41. The cast is trimmed around the toes to allow inspection and exercises.

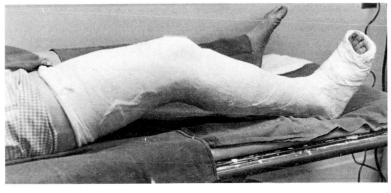

Figure 4-42. Completed long leg cast.

knee is usually placed in approximately 20 to 30 degrees of flexion.

Cylinder Cast. The cylinder cast is applied to the lower extremity from below the hip to above the ankle and is primarily used to immobilize the knee, usually in extension (Fig. 4-43). The biggest practical problem after application of a cylinder cast is that it will tend to shuck up and down on the extremity, rubbing the Achilles tendon above the ankle and causing discomfort. A skin slough over the Achilles tendon is to be avoided *at all costs*. Attention to some small details will minimize this problem. The following method is helpful to prevent the cast from shucking up and down: paint or spray the skin with benzoin (Fig. 4-44); next, roll on stockinette (usually 3- or 4-inch). This will adhere to the benzoin and the skin, and the soft cotton padding is then applied as previously discussed (Fig. 4-45). Several extra turns of the soft cotton roll are made at the distal end of the cast to pad the area of the heel cord, as well as below the hip to pad the top edge of the cast. While the plaster is still in a ductile state the cast is rubbed just above the femoral condyles, in an attempt to mold it to the contour of the femur and prevent it from shucking up and down. The cylinder cast should stop where there is still some muscle tissue present in the heel cord area, just above the prominent subcutaneous heel cord. Before the final roll of plaster is applied, the stockinette at the distal end of the extremity is turned back and incorporated into the cast (Figs. 4-46, 4-47). This suspends the cast by the adhesiveness of the stockinette to the skin, which has been painted with benzoin, and will usually minimize the shucking action of the cast even after atrophy has occurred. Occasionally a suspender or sling is used around the pelvis and hip and attached to a cylinder cast if shucking is a problem, or the cylinder may need to be changed.

Casts may be applied with gentle pressure to accomplish correction of a deformity; for example, a clubfoot cast. In general, the extremity is manipulated and held in the maximum position of correction while the cast is applied. Gentle, firm corrective pressure can be exerted at the time the cast is applied as long as the cast is rubbed carefully and meticulously to prevent pressure points. Casts are occasionally cut and wedged to gain further correction. For example, a snug, smooth cast may be placed on a clubfoot, molding it gently into a position of maximum correction. After the foot has been maintained for 7 to 10 days in the position of maximum correction, the muscles, ligaments, and joints have usually gently stretched out and more correction is obtainable. By cutting the cast and taking out a portion in such a fashion that after removal of this portion the cast edges can be brought together, the correction can be increased. The edges of the cut cast must be crimped with a cast bender so that they do not cut into the skin when the corrective position is achieved. Too much correction should not be attempted at any one time.

During the application of any cast, when stockinette has been placed on the extremity it should be turned back onto the cast and the final roll of plaster at the upper and lower ends of the cast is applied to hold down the loose ends of the

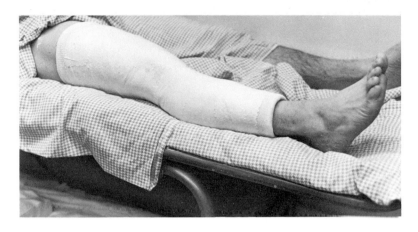

Figure 4-43. Completed cylinder cast.

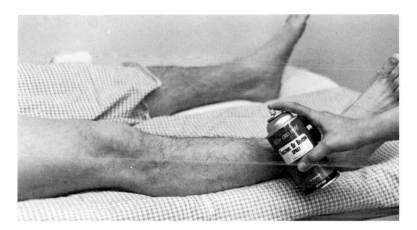

Figure 4-44. Benzoin applied to leg.

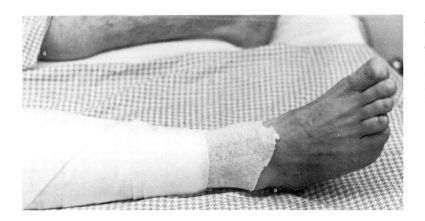

Figure 4-45. Soft cotton padding applied at the distal end of the cylinder to protect the Achilles tendon.

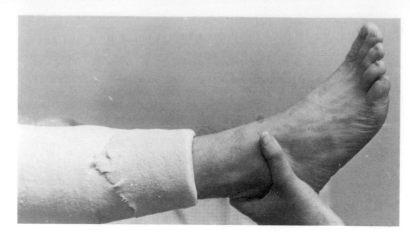

*Figure 4-46.
Stockinette
turned back into
the cast.*

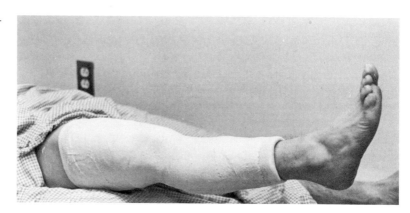

*Figure 4-47. Com-
pleted cylinder
cast.*

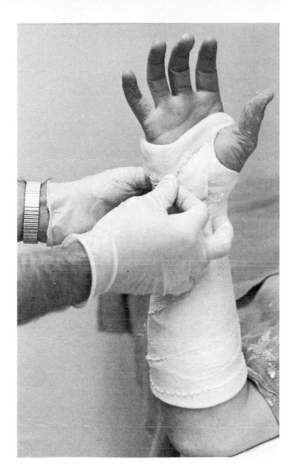

Figure 4-48.
Stockinette
turned back into
the cast.

stockinette (Fig. 4-48). This increases patient comfort and improves the appearance of the cast.

When trimming the cast is necessary, a plaster knife (Fig. 4-49) is used to trim a soft cast (approximately 2 minutes after the cast has first become firm), and a plaster saw if the plaster has set (usually about 10 minutes after application).

After application of a cast a pillow may be needed to support the extremity. Never use a rubber pillow, since it does not allow the heat to dissipate.

The excess plaster should be cleaned off the patient.

A sling or crutches may be needed for support, depending on the type of cast applied.

Splints. Many different types of splints may be used: wood, metal, plastic, or leather. A plaster splint is a partial cast; it

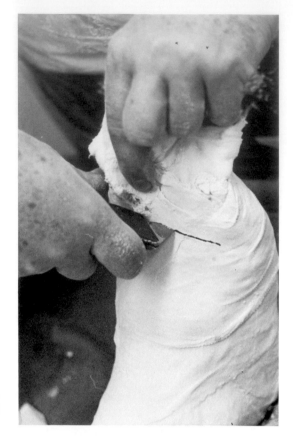

Figure 4-49. Trimming the cast with a cast knife.

may be made from the front or back half of a cast, or from layers of plaster (Fig. 4-50).

Splints are often used when a temporary support for a joint or extremity is needed that will allow for swelling or for easy removal of the dressing or splint. Prepackaged splints are available. However, if the splint is to be fabricated, plaster in its dry state is rolled back and forth to the desired length and then dipped into warm water; it is fan-folded and the excess water is removed, and then it is rubbed together to make a solid splint. While the splint is still damp, it can be backed with soft cotton padding before wrapping it on the extremity with an elastic bandage; this prevents it from adhering to the dressing and makes it much easier to remove than if the raw, damp plaster is applied directly to the dressings and the elastic bandage wrapped over the plaster. Another way to back a splint is to put the plaster in a stockinette. Forearm and knee splints can be made up in stockinette and placed on the emergency room or office shelves; then they can be dipped into

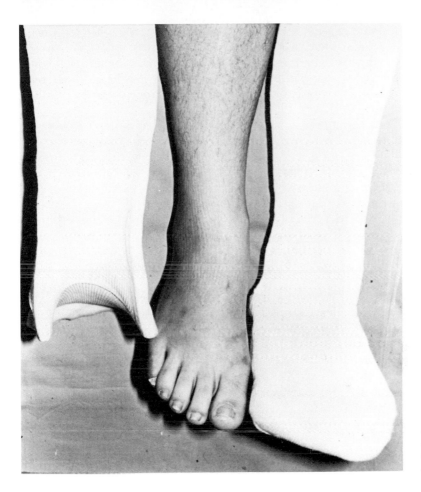

Figure 4-50. Short leg cast, bivalved and used for a splint.

the water in the stockinette and applied when needed. Leg splints are usually made out of approximately 6 to 8 thicknesses of 5- or 6-inch plaster, long enough to extend from below the hip to the distal third of the leg; they are used to support the knee. The most commonly used arm splints are cock-up wrist splints. These can be constructed of approximately 8 to 10 layers of 3- or 4-inch plaster extending from just proximal to the palmar crease to 2 to 3 inches below the elbow.

PATIENT INSTRUCTIONS. Patients must be instructed not only in the care of the cast but also in the recognition of those signs and symptoms that should be reported to the physician.

Instructions to the patient should include *avoiding* the following: physical abuse of the cast; allowing it to get wet; removing the padding from beneath the cast; scratching underneath it with any object (this may cut or abrade the skin and cause infection); placing or dropping a foreign object under the cast (these can cause pressure areas); weight bearing on a green cast (48 to 72 hours must be allowed for the cast to completely harden); and keeping the cast covered with a plastic or rubber wrapping that prevents evaporation of moisture.

Appropriate instructions must be given concerning elevation of the extremity. This is especially important for the first 24 to 48 hours following fracture. Elevation *higher than the level of the heart* must be stressed.

Joints above and below the cast must be exercised in order to prevent stiffness as well as maintain muscle tone.

Ice applied directly over a fracture site for the first 24 hours will reduce swelling. Any plastic bag (even an old bread bag) may be used to hold the ice; however, it should be covered with a washcloth or towel to keep the cast from becoming wet.

The signs and symptoms that the patient should report to the physician include increasing pain, unrelieved by the normal medication; moderate swelling associated with pain and discoloration of the toes or fingers; pain on motion, especially passive motion; and burning or tingling underneath the cast.

NURSING CARE. Personnel involved in the care of an individual in a cast must always remember that a cast is rigid; with swelling, pressure constriction of an extremity may occur with grave complications (Fig. 4-51). Because of the inability to view the extremity, neurovascular checks of the distal part must be done *as needed* to document the integrity of neurovascular function. One must always be suspicious; observation, recognition, and prompt action for neurovascular complications must be an integral part of the care plan.

A firm mattress as well as pillows should be used as a supportive measure for the individual in a cast.

Nursing actions should include use of a heat lamp, bed cradle, or hair dryer to speed the drying process; daily inspection of all visible skin; and use of 70 percent alcohol on all skin that comes in contact with the cast. If stockinette has not been used in the application of the cast and turned back over the exposed plaster edges, the edges may be petaled. This is accomplished by covering the edges with moleskin or adhesive tape. For patients in body casts, the perineal area must be protected with waterproof material, the head of the bed should be elevated when a bedpan is used, and frequent turning is necessary; however, turning must not be done by the bar at the legs of the cast.

When ambulation is begun, a sling will be needed to support an arm cast. Patients in short or long leg casts will require crutches or a walker; usually three-point gait, either weight bearing or non-weight bearing, will be used.

190

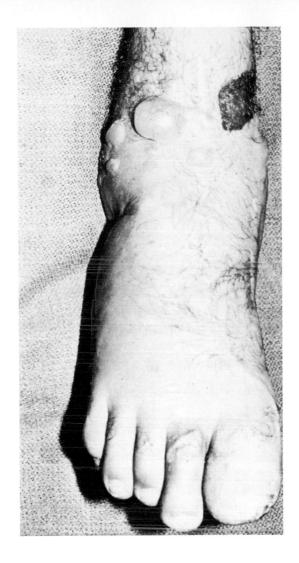

Figure 4-51. Circulatory damage from swelling in the cast

REMOVAL OF A CAST. A cast is removed for the following reasons: when it is no longer necessary for immobilization; in order to change the position of the extremity in the cast; when an x-ray is needed to see healing at the fracture site (x-rays are generally taken through plaster to check alignment only); and when the cast is damaged through misuse or length of time in place.

Equipment needed for cast removal is as follows: electric cast saw, plain or with vacuum; cast spreaders, manual or spring; a cast knife; and bandage scissors.

The procedure should be explained to the patient, and one should emphasize that the saw does not cut the skin because the blade vibrates rather than rotates. However, the operator must remember that if prolonged pressure is applied with the

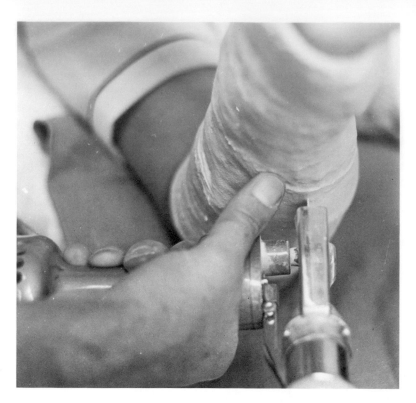

*Figure 4-52. Re-
moval of the cast
using a saw.*

cast saw, particularly in an area with very little subcutaneous
padding and fat (the most dangerous areas are the bony prominences of the ankle, the head of the fibula, and the wrist),
even the pressure and heat of the vibrating blade can cut the
skin. Touch the blade lightly to your hand or your arm to re-
assure the patient.

The cast is supported by the operator's hand or by pillows.
The saw is held with the four fingers around the handle. The
thumb touches the plaster before the blade does, and acts as a
stop. Starting at either end of one side of the cast, the saw is
applied with pressure and control on the plaster until slack is
felt (Fig. 4-52). The saw is then quickly removed and placed
on the next section. This procedure is repeated until both
sides of the cast have been cut.

The cast spreaders are then used to spread the cast apart.
This is accomplished by inserting the working end of the
spreader into the area that has been cut by the saw and
squeezing the handles together until the cast separates. This is
repeated until the cast is separated in all areas.

The scissors are then used to cut the stockinette or soft cotton padding (Fig. 4-53). Bandage scissors should always be
used to avoid cutting the patient. Never use sharp-pointed
scissors.

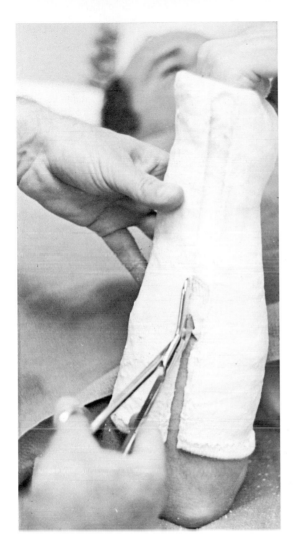

Figure 4-53. Cutting the padding beneath the cast.

The top shell of the cast is then removed while the affected part is gently and firmly supported. The patient must be told that, although the extremity may feel strange on removal from the cast, with careful handling it will not be injured. The bottom shell of the cast is removed with continuing support of the affected part. The skin which was covered by the cast may be flaky, and the muscles and joints will be sore and stiff.

Never wash the skin if a second cast is to be applied.

This same procedure is followed when *bivalving* a cast; however, the two halves are left in place and the stockinette or padding may or may not be cut, depending on the physician's

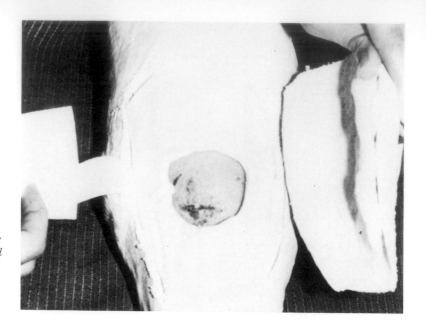

Figure 4-54. The cast is windowed and the skin and window are appropriately padded.

instructions. The halves may be held in place with an elastic bandage wrap, Velcro straps, or adhesive tape.

When a cast is bivalved to relieve edema it should be cut along its entire length, spread slightly, and the circular bandage beneath it cut, unless other instructions are given.

Cutting out a piece of the plaster around an incision or a pressure area is called windowing (Fig. 4-54). The plaster is cut in the same manner as previously described and a window is removed using the cast spreaders. The soft wrapping beneath may or may not be cut depending on the purpose of the window. The piece of cast is always replaced with tape, plaster, or an elastic bandage wrap. If this is not done, swelling of the area through the window may occur.

General Preoperative Nursing Care

Prior to surgery, the patient should have an understanding of those devices and treatments which will be necessary during the postoperative phase. This may be accomplished by the following nursing actions: demonstration or explanation of the type of device, such as cast, traction or splint, to be used postoperatively; instruction in the planned postoperative exercise program; instruction in the appropriate respiratory therapy, coughing and deep breathing, blow bottle, or intermediate positive pressure breathing; and, if surgery is to be performed on the lower extremity, instruction in the use of pelvic lift to facilitate postoperative use of the bedpan, back care, and bed making.

An explanation of the preliminary diagnostic studies or procedures must be given to the patient. These usually include laboratory studies, x-rays, and in many instances an electrocardiogram.

Since the chance of postoperative infection is minimized by reducing the number of skin bacteria, the operative and surrounding area is usually scrubbed with a bacteriostatic or antiseptic solution several times prior to surgery. Although many patients will have begun this practice prior to admission to the hospital, assistance should be given during the preoperative period to ensure the adequacy of the scrub. During this procedure the skin should be inspected for cuts, abrasions, or infected areas; if present, these should be reported to the physician. This same area is shaved immediately preoperatively, care being taken not to cut or abrade the skin, which would increase the chance of infection. Orthopedic procedures have been canceled for this very reason.

Most patients undergoing major surgery of the back, hip, or lower extremity will be given an enema preoperatively because of the diminished peristalsis anticipated in the immediate postoperative period.

When surgery is to be performed on the hip or lower extremity, crutches or a walker will be required postoperatively for ambulation. The patient should be fitted with the appropriate assistive gait device and instructed in the anticipated gait pattern preoperatively, to facilitate postoperative ambulation.

Following major orthopedic surgery, bleeding from the wound is anticipated; therefore, wound suction is frequently used to decrease the possibility of a hematoma. The patient and his or her family should be prepared for seeing this apparatus at the wound site postoperatively.

Postoperative bleeding through the cast (Fig. 4-55) should be anticipated and the patient must be alerted to this before surgery. It should be explained to the patient that a small amount of bleeding will diffuse widely through the exterior of a cast and need not be viewed with alarm.

Information should be provided which will enable the patient to better understand the anticipated surgery as well as the anticipated goals of the procedure.

Blood replacement is necessary following many major orthopedic surgical procedures. The patient should have an un-

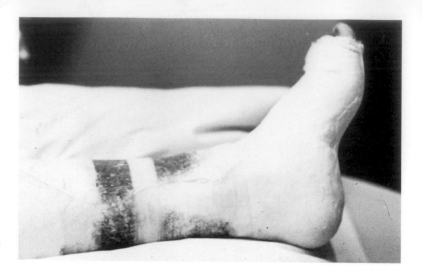

*Figure 4-55.
Bleeding through
the cast postoper-
atively.*

derstanding of this necessity as well as of the hospital's
routine concerning this procedure.

Patients with rheumatoid arthritis and those who have received steroid therapy in the past are usually given steroids in
the immediate preoperative period. The physician must be
alerted to any patient history of steroid therapy.

The surgical and recovery room suites are very frightening
to those unfamiliar with their routines. The patient should
know what to expect during the preanesthetic and recovery
room periods.

General Postoperative Nursing Care

The long-term nursing goal for any patient following surgery
should be to provide nursing care that will allow return, after
rehabilitation, to the maximal functional level consistent with
the surgery to be performed.

General postoperative nursing care for orthopedic patients
is the same as for other surgical patients in regard to skin
care, intake and output records, possible abdominal distension or urine retention, pneumonia, and the preventive measures necessary for the other possible complications of immobility. (Complications that are known hazards to the
orthopedic patient are discussed later in this chapter.)

Often, following major orthopedic surgery, a wound suction
apparatus is inserted in anticipation of further blood loss into
the tissues. Use of wound suction lessens the chances of

wound hematoma. The tubing from the wound may be connected to its own bellows or to a low suction device. The drainage fluid should be emptied every eight hours and recorded on a separate output sheet. If the fluid is excessive or bright red, the physician should be notified immediately. The suction apparatus is usually removed 48 hours after operation.

When surgery has been performed for an infection, wound suction-irrigation may be used for some time postoperatively. Two to 4 tubes may be inserted directly into the wound; 1 or 2 being used for irrigation and 1 or 2 for suction. The tubes designated as the out, or suction, tubes will be connected to suction, either a portable unit or low wall suction. The tubes designated as the in, infusion, and irrigation tubes will be connected to intravenous or irrigation fluids containing massive doses of antibiotics. The rate of infusion will be determined by the physician; however, it is the responsibility of the nurse to maintain this therapy and accurately record the infusion as well as the drainage (suction).

Should the tubing become clogged it may be flushed with 10 ml of normal saline, or the physician may allow the tubes to be alternated (infusion tubes become suction tubes, and vice versa) at intervals or when they become clogged. The incidence of clogging is decreased when wound suction is maintained continuously.

A separate intake and output sheet must be kept for wound suction-irrigation.

NURSING CARE FOLLOWING SURGERY OF THE HIP. In postoperative management of the hip, the following basic principles apply to all patients: Maintain the involved leg in abduction, avoid extremes of rotation and acute hip flexion, and handle the leg gently.

Each case is of course different, depending on the surgical approach to the hip, the type of surgery done (nail, prosthesis, or arthroplasty), and the surgeon's preference in the postoperative management of his or her patients. Ideally, these basic principles are taught to all the appropriate personnel, so that the patient will receive expert care 24 hours a day. Often, in efforts to teach other personnel, the issue is confused by cautions that "this patient can" or "this patient cannot." The attitude should be that there are basic principles in the care of all patients following surgery of the hip.

There are some very real reasons for maintaining the involved leg in abduction. With the leg in neutral position, the femoral head is well seated in the socket; with the leg in the abducted position, the femoral head is even better seated in the socket; but with the leg in adduction, the femoral head may begin to dislocate from the socket or the nail may begin to pull out. Since adduction is a relatively unstable position, the leg should be kept in a position of abduction at all times. This position is accomplished through the use of an abduction pillow, split Russell traction, balanced suspension, two pillows kept between the legs, or any other commonly used abduction device. If the patient is in traction but not in enough abduction because of body size, simply add a longer side bar to the bed. Be aware that patients will adduct by themselves by sliding down in bed and bringing the shoulders over to the opposite side of the bed. Patients must be taught the appropriate position: hips and shoulders in the middle of the bed, involved leg out to the side.

The safest position for the leg in regard to rotation depends on the type of surgical approach that was used. In general, the safest position for the hip is neutral to slight external rotation. To maintain this position it may be necessary to use a folded towel or sandbag with the pillow, or a trochanteric roll under the hip operated on. Abduction is to be maintained during turning, and extremes of rotation should be avoided.

Acute hip flexion must also be avoided, since this position can cause posterior dislocation. After prosthetic replacement or total hip arthroplasty, for several days postoperatively the head of the bed should not be elevated more than 45 degrees. When postoperative exercise of the leg is begun, and certainly when the patient begins to be ambulatory, the hip is not to be flexed beyond 90 degrees.

Muscle spasms cause pain and irritation to the joint. Do not touch a patient's leg after operation before explaining what you are going to do. Any patient's hip can be moved postoperatively if it is handled gently. Remember that if you feel confident in managing the patient's leg, the patient will have confidence in you.

The general nursing care of the orthopedic patient is the same as that for all patients who have had major surgery. The surgeon assumes that the patient's hygienic needs will be met. Basic nursing care measures are used to prevent thrombophlebitis and emboli, respiratory complications, and gastrointestinal dysfunction, and to avert genitourinary complications. Although the hip is fragile in many cases, the surgeon does realize that routine nursing care activities must be performed.

With the surgeon's approval, the patient may be turned to the opposite side for back care and bed making. If the patient cannot be turned, pelvic lift may be utilized for these functions.

A simple exercise sling is used to assist the patient in gaining hip and knee motion. When there is some muscular control of the hip and the soft tissues are sufficiently healed, use of the sling is an excellent way for a patient to start moving the hip or prosthesis.

With the sling positioned under the knee, the patient can pull on the handle and give himself gentle, assisted hip and knee flexion. If the sling is positioned under the calf of the affected leg, the patient can pull on the handle and lift the leg off the bed, giving himself active, assisted hip abduction and adduction as well as knee extension. If the patient does this by using his own muscles, assisted by the sling, it is active, assisted abduction and adduction of the hip. If the hip motion is to be strictly passive, the patient can hold the leg off the bed by pulling on the handle of the knee sling, but a nurse or a therapist will then have to gently abduct and adduct the leg as the physician has prescribed. When the patient has a knee sling under the knee and pulls on it without using his leg muscles, he is getting strictly passive hip and knee flexion. Remember that an arthroplasty of the hip is never adducted past the midline, as the adducted position is relatively unstable. The motion of the adduction is usually carried out from the safe abducted position toward, but not past, the midline.

The timing of progressive ambulation will usually depend on the type of surgery performed and on the physician's preference.

When the patient is allowed to begin sitting on the side of the bed, the best way to accomplish this, in general, is as follows: The patient assumes a sitting position, facing toward the operative side. The leg is cradled in slight abduction by the nurse. The knee is carefully allowed to bend as the patient sits on the edge of the bed, and the foot is allowed to rest comfortably on the floor. In this position, the hip is protected from acute flexion. It is often helpful for the patient to gently exercise the feet and ankles with both feet on the floor, by carefully pushing up on the toes and then rocking back on the heels. The hip is also kept in abduction.

The next phase of progression is supervised standing by the bed with a walker. The bed is raised high enough to allow the patient to slide out with ease. At first postural hypotension may be a problem, but if the patient is instructed in tiptoe exercise (rocking back and forth on the heels and toes) this exercise will often facilitate the return of blood to the cardiovascular system and rapidly overcome the problem of hypotension. The patient is allowed to put the involved leg on the floor, but guided to allow the hands and the normal hip to bear most of the weight. The amount of supportable weight is determined by the physician. The bed is lowered when the patient is getting back into bed. When the patient can stand by the bed in the walker comfortably and confidently, he is usually allowed to begin walking carefully in the room. A partial weight bearing gait is usually appropriate, and the patient is instructed to use the involved leg in a normal gait pattern. Progressive walking for short periods of time in the hospital hall is then instituted. It is generally better for a patient to walk for a short time with a correct stance and gait pattern than to walk for a longer distance with a limp and poor posture.

Crutches are used when the patient's ability and confidence warrant. Often, an elderly patient may require the stability of a walker indefinitely.

In some cases, the patient will only be allowed to feel the floor with the foot or to touch down, essentially bearing no weight on the extremity. In other cases, the patient may be allowed to use the walker only for transfer from bed to chair, bearing no weight on the involved hip. The patient usually is allowed to sit on a chair at about the same time he begins walking with a walker in the room. The patient should always sit in a high chair, never a low one. Chairs with arms are preferable. An elevated commode with arms should be used for patients over 5 feet, 4 inches tall.

It is important to allow each patient to progress at his or her own pace, bearing in mind that patients with bilateral hip involvement or rheumatoid arthritis and multiple joint involvement will require a longer time and more help in their convalescence. The rate of progression of weight bearing, the duration and type of external support, and the pace of resumption of normal activities must be decided by the orthopedic surgeon. Only he is aware of the many factors influencing his decision (condition of the patient's bone, type of procedure, technical difficulties at the time of surgery, the patient's personality, and his own philosophy).

NURSING CARE FOLLOWING SURGERY OF THE FEMUR. One to 2 units of blood may be lost into the thigh postoperatively without any external signs of bleeding; therefore, patients must be continuously assessed for signs of blood loss.

The leg that was operated on should be placed in a position of comfort, usually slight hip and knee flexion and slight external rotation. Often the leg will be uncomfortable during the early postoperative phase if it is in a position of extreme external rotation, as the skin over the buttock becomes stuck to the linens of the bed. This may be relieved by having the patient use pelvic lift while the nurse places a hand under the affected buttock, gently drawing the skin and tissues laterally. This allows the leg to lie in the more normal position of slight external rotation. A soft trochanteric roll is often used to prevent excessive external rotation. Frequently, a change in position of the extremity promotes comfort. The patient should be told that this can be accomplished without injury to the extremity.

An elastic bandage wrap may be used around the thigh to compress and support the tissues. If edema occurs distal to the wrap, an elastic stocking or elastic bandage wrapping of the entire extremity may be necessary to prevent venous stasis. Neurovascular checks are important in the distal portion of the extremity to detect any compromise from pressure and swelling at the surgical site. Gentle, active exercises of the foot and ankle will improve circulation in the leg and decrease distal edema.

The patient may be turned to the opposite side for back care and comfort, resting the involved extremity on two pillows to avoid the strained position of adduction and internal rotation.

The patient can be taught very gentle, active assisted extension and flexion exercises for the knee to be done within the limits of pain several times daily, even in the acute postoperative phase. Muscles are retracted and transected at the time of surgery; therefore, these exercises should be assisted with a knee sling or the nurse's hand.

The patient can usually be mobilized within a few days of surgery. This will depend on the stability of the femur as well as on the patient's discomfort. He may need assistance in handling his leg getting in and out of bed. This may be accomplished by his tucking the foot of the uninvolved extremity underneath the ankle of the leg which was operated on, thereby supporting the extremity, or another person may support the leg during this transfer. Whether or not the patient will be allowed to rest the extremity on the floor when standing with crutches or a walker, and how much weight may be borne, will depend on the surgeon's evaluation of the stability of the femur.

NURSING CARE FOLLOWING SURGERY OF THE KNEE. Regardless of the type of surgery performed, usually the involved knee will be more comfortable in a position of some flexion, since this allows for swelling in the knee joint and relaxes the posterior capsule of the knee. For this reason, some knee flexion may be allowed during the postoperative phase, as long as the knee is not in a flexed position at all times; it should be extended for at least part of the time during the day.

If the knee is wrapped with an elastic bandage, edema may occur distally. This can be prevented or minimized by a distal compression wrapping and foot and ankle exercises.

Severe pain occurring in the early postoperative phase usually indicates bleeding into the joint. This pain is relieved by analgesics, ice caps, and gentle quadriceps setting exercises, but if the effusion is persistent and quite painful the knee joint may need to be aspirated by the surgeon.

The knee may be splinted to maintain it in a position of extension. If the splint may be opened for comfort several times daily, this will be specified by appropriate orders. The extremity may also be in a cylinder or long leg cast depending on the type of surgery performed.

In general, the patient should begin straightening the knee, thereby setting the quadricep muscle, as soon as pain permits, unless there has been some particular surgery that contraindicates this (for example, repairs of the quadriceps tendon or patella). This setting exercise should be demonstrated on the normal extremity before it is attempted on the involved side. It may be helpful for the patient to perform this exercise on both extremities at the same time. A gentle attempt to actively extend and flex the knee just a few degrees, done several times daily, will generally decrease the effusion, improve circulation, and increase comfort.

During the postoperative phase, when it is imperative for the patient to begin active straight leg raising, be sure that he or she is encouraged to keep the patella straight up as this exercise is done. Frequently a patient will lift the leg without contracting the quadriceps by externally rotating the knee, thereby substituting the medial collateral ligament for the quadriceps.

When the patient begins to walk he or she will need assistance with the affected extremity. The patient should be taught to use the uninvolved extremity (tucking the foot under the ankle of the involved extremity) to support the side that was operated on. However, assistance may be needed in supporting the extremity for the first several times when getting in and out of bed.

Walking and weight bearing are allowed according to the physician's orders, depending on the type of surgery performed. When there is no loss of ligamentous stability and bony strength of the joint, such as in a meniscectomy, weight bearing within the limits of pain is allowed.

An assistive gait device, such as crutches or a walker, will be needed during the beginning ambulation period. The length of time these are to be used will depend on the surgery performed.

NURSING CARE FOLLOWING SURGERY OF THE TIBIA. Much of the postoperative nursing care will depend on whether the extremity is in a short or a long cast or in a soft compression dressing. Neurovascular checks are a must.

In the immediate postoperative period the extremity must be elevated constantly to minimize swelling, thereby prevent-

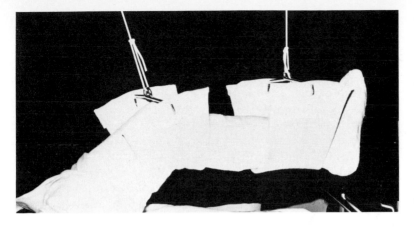

Figure 4-56. Sling elevation for a fractured lower extremity.

ing compartment syndrome. The extremity must be supported with pillows or slings, which allow it to be parallel to the bed (Fig. 4-56).

If the extremity is in a short cast or soft compression dressing, elevation will require flexing the knee and placing the lower part of the leg on pillows. If the foot is simply elevated, the knee is placed in a position of excessive extension that will be most uncomfortable. Several times daily the leg should be fully extended to avoid flexion contracture of the knee.

Even with the extremity in a cast, foot and ankle exercises, as allowed by the cast, should be encouraged within the limits of pain.

Ambulation will require the use of some assistive gait device, such as crutches or a walker. Weight bearing will be as ordered by the physician.

NURSING CARE FOLLOWING SURGERY OF THE FOOT AND ANKLE. Elevation to reduce swelling and promote comfort is indicated in the early postoperative phase and may be accomplished with the use of pillows or slings. When slings are used, they should be placed so as to avoid peroneal nerve pressure. If pillows are used, they should support the entire leg below the knee, allowing the knee to flex and thus avoiding undue stress on the posterior capsule. The knee should be fully extended several times daily.

If the foot tends to drop into equinus, a support should be utilized at the foot of the bed to maintain a neutral position.

If it is sensitive, the leg should be protected from the bed linen by use of an appropriate bed cradle.

Neurovascular checks of the toes are necessary.

Active range of motion exercises distal to the site of surgery should be done several times daily within the limits of pain.

The use of crutches or a walker will generally be required for walking.

NURSING CARE FOLLOWING SURGERY OF THE SHOULDER. Usually the shoulder will be placed in a position of rest postoperatively, with the arm at the side, the forearm across the chest, and the elbow bent 90 degrees. This will place the shoulder in internal rotation, the stable position for many shoulder injuries or repairs. In general, the shoulder is more comfortable if a small rolled sheet is placed under the humerus, lifting the shaft slightly forward. Occasionally the humerus will be supported postoperatively in a position of abduction in an abduction splint or side arm traction.

The dressing should be observed for bleeding. Neurovascular checks must be done to ascertain the neurovascular status of the arm.

If dressings permit, the axilla may be cleaned once or twice daily and a clean pad with talcum powder on it inserted.

Regardless of the type of postoperative dressing, some motion in the joint will make it more comfortable and frequent changes of position, even though slight, enhance the patient's comfort.

Exercises of the fingers and wrist within the limits of pain should be encouraged. Unless otherwise ordered, very gentle shoulder shrugging may be permitted, to give a little motion to the joint. When it is not too painful, gentle isometric setting exercises for the muscles of the shoulder and arm will prevent a sensation of subluxation and tension in the shoulder.

When the patient is in a sitting position, the weight of the arm will tend to give a feeling of pull on the shoulder. This is relieved by a sling that supports the weight of the arm or by having the patient support the forearm and elbow with the unaffected extremity.

Following any type of upper extremity surgery there is bleeding into the tissues postoperatively. Ecchymosis and discoloration will normally be present during the early postoperative period. This will be manifested by some soreness and discoloration extending into the pectoral (breast) area and down the arm, even into the forearm and fingers. It should be explained to the patient that this is not unusual and is to be expected. When soreness is caused by this extravasation of blood into the muscle and fascial planes, warm applications for 30 minutes, 4 times daily, give relief.

NURSING CARE FOLLOWING SURGERY OF THE HUMERUS. The postoperative care of the humerus is the same as after that of the shoulder, with a few exceptions.

After surgery on the humeral shaft, a patient is often most comfortable in a sitting or semisitting position, so that the weight of the arm (with the wrist being supported in a collar and cuff arrangement around the neck) tends to align the humerus and make it comfortable.

When the surgeon allows, the arm can be carefully slipped out of the sling to allow active assisted range of motion exercises to the elbow several times daily.

NURSING CARE FOLLOWING SURGERY OF THE ELBOW. The extremity will usually be immobilized in some type of splint or cast and must be elevated in the immediate postoperative period.

Neurovascular checks must be performed routinely. The nurse must always be alert to the signs of compartment syndrome following surgery.

Attention should be directed toward preserving shoulder motion as well as wrist and finger motion. The shoulder should be circumducted several times daily through the use of pendulum exercises or physical assistance.

At some time in the postoperative period, the arm may be removed from the splint several times daily for gentle, guided, active assisted range of motion exercises.

NURSING CARE FOLLOWING SURGERY OF THE FOREARM. The extremity usually is immobilized in a splint or plaster cast. The arm should be elevated higher than the heart.

Attention must be given to the neurovascular status of the fingers.

Motion in the fingers as well as the shoulder should be encouraged.

NURSING CARE FOLLOWING SURGERY OF THE WRIST AND HAND. Following surgery of the hand or wrist, the forearm and hand will be placed in some type of compression dressing with or without splints.

The wrist and hand should be elevated, and this is usually most satisfactorily accomplished by use of some type of sling such as a Columbia. Care should be taken to allow the elbow to rest on the bed so that the patient does not have the feeling that the arm is being pulled and suspended by the affected wrist and hand. The sling is used simply to maintain the hand and wrist in an elevated position.

Encourage very gentle finger motion unless the surgeon orders otherwise. Have the patient "play the piano" for 5 minutes out of every hour during the waking hours.

NURSING CARE FOLLOWING SURGERY OF THE CERVICAL SPINE. The patient will be put in skeletal traction of the cervical spine if a precarious situation exists. Appropriate nursing measures for the patient in cervical traction should be followed.

For other types of cervical spinal surgery, when there is no marked instability of the cervical spine the patient will usually be treated postoperatively in a soft or rigid collar that will maintain the neck in neutral or slight extension and avoid extremes of rotation and flexion. In most cases, if the patient is reassured and allowed to rest quietly in a recumbent position the collar can be gently loosened for comfort and skin care and then replaced.

These patients must be observed for signs of respiratory distress. Such signs warrant removal of the collar or brace for relief and proper assessment of possible hematoma formation in the wound. The surgeon must be notified immediately of any signs of respiratory distress.

NURSING CARE FOLLOWING SURGERY OF THE BACK. Positioning is important postoperatively to reduce stress on the back, as well as to decrease pain. The incidence of wound hematoma is reduced when the patient lies flat on his back for several hours postoperatively. Positioning should be accomplished by employing the log-rolling technique. Log rolling is accomplished by having the patient turn his body as a unit, keeping the hips and shoulders in a straight line, with the knees slightly flexed. This position should be supported with pillows at the back and hips and between the legs.

Some patients will be allowed to turn themselves as soon as pain permits; this is determined by the physician. The use of the trapeze also depends on the physician's directions.

The degree of elevation of the head of the bed is determined by the physician.

When the patient becomes ambulatory, a corset or brace may be used to assist the abdominal and back muscles in supporting the spine. An undershirt worn under a corset or brace is helpful in protecting the skin and areas over the bony prominences.

An elevated commode seat is very helpful to these patients.

In general, these patients should not sit for long periods of time.

Modified general bed exercises may be instituted immediately postoperatively, but the specific exercise program for strengthening the abdominal and back muscles will be ordered by the physician.

These principles apply to patients who have had disc surgery and to most spinal fusion patients. The rapidity of mobilization, the type of bracing, and specific nursing care depend on the extent of the fusion and on the specific instructions of the orthopedic surgeon.

The nursing care of the postoperative scoliosis patient may be quite complicated. Usually the fusion is extensive and internal spinal instrumentation may have been utilized. The patient generally has to undergo a long period of recumbency with the usual positioning and log-rolling techniques, followed by gradual ambulation in appropriate special braces. It is desirable for the orthopedic nurse to be familiar with the special techniques and intricacies of management of the post-operative scoliosis patient and with the devices utilized in his care. The interested reader should consult a text which deals specifically with surgery and nursing care for scoliosis.

NURSING CARE OF THE AMPUTEE. Following an amputation the patient must have not only physical support, but emotional support as well. Active participation in his rehabilitation is of the utmost importance.

Immediately postoperatively, watch for signs of hemorrhage. Some oozing from the stump is to be expected and the dressing may be reinforced; however, should hemorrhage occur, apply direct pressure to the stump immediately by means of a firm Ace bandage wrap, hand pressure, or both. The foot of the bed should be raised to elevate the lower extremity stump.

To prevent contracture deformities, the patient should be encouraged to turn from side to side, to move the stump, and to perform range of motion exercises for the joint above the amputation several times daily. The patient should also be placed in the prone position twice daily.

The care plan should include those muscle strengthening and balancing exercises necessary to increase the patient's mobility.

Stump care includes use of an elastic wrap, stump conditioning exercises, massages, and cleanliness.

The patient may experience phantom limb sensation (the feeling that the limb is still present) or phantom pain (painful sensation). This sensation or pain may or may not occur postoperatively and may last for only a few hours or for years. The patient should be told that this is not abnormal.

Whether there is to be immediate or delayed prosthetic fitting will be determined by the physician.

Complications Frequently Seen in Orthopedic Nursing
The nurse caring for the orthopedic patient must be aware of those occurrences which may pose a hazard to that patient. Not only should the nurse be knowledgeable concerning the usual signs and symptoms of these complications, but she or he should also understand any preventive measures and the usual treatment. The nursing care plan must have incorporated concurrently and recurrently all nursing actions necessary for the anticipation, recognition, and treatment of these complications.

THROMBOPHLEBITIS. Thrombophlebitis is intravascular clotting which may be caused by venous stasis, hypercoagulation, or endothelial damage, the primary factor being slowing of the circulation and damage to the vessel wall. This complication is most frequently seen in the lower extremities.

Prevention. Whenever an individual is confined to bed venous return is slowed down considerably, partly because of the decrease in muscular activity of the lower extremities which normally pumps the blood from the legs back to the heart. Nursing intervention should be directed toward those activities which will increase the activity of the lower extremities, increasing blood flow and thereby preventing venous stasis.

Foot and ankle exercises should begin preoperatively or immediately after injury. These should be done frequently when the patient is up in a chair as well as when in bed. Dependent positions of the legs should be avoided. General bed exercises should be encouraged. The patient should begin walking as early as possible.

Antiembolic stockings have been shown to be effective in increasing the venous velocity in the legs. When used, however, the stockings should be removed for one hour every 8 hours and the calf carefully inspected for edema or tenderness. They must be carefully fitted and prevented from rolling up at the top, blocking venous return.

Heparin, Coumadin, aspirin, and low-molecular-weight dextran are sometimes used in the prophylactic drug management of thrombophlebitis.

Recognition. The clinical manifestations of thrombophlebitis include calf tenderness, edema, increased temperature or redness of the extremity, and elevated temperature. Homan's sign (pain in the calf on dorsiflexion) should be evaluated every 8 hours. Increased calf circumference of greater than one-half to one inch may be indicative of thrombophlebitis. In the early course of thrombophlebitis venous pressures can be taken; the venous pressure will be higher in the unaffected leg.

Phlebography, ultrasonic flow detection, and isotope studies are helpful in the diagnosis.

PULMONARY EMBOLUS. Pulmonary embolism is the obstruction of one or more pulmonary arteries, most commonly caused by a clot (thrombus) originating somewhere in the venous system. The thrombus usually originates in the deep veins of the legs or pelvis; however, it may come from the veins in the arm or, rarely, from the right side of the heart. If there is resultant damage to the lung tissue the term *pulmonary infarction* is used.

Prevention. Because most emboli originate in the veins of the lower extremities or pelvic area due to stasis of venous circulation, all preventive measures discussed in thrombophlebitis apply. Remember, *the prevention of thrombophlebitis is usually the prevention of pulmonary emboli.*

High-risk patients are those patients with a history of thrombophlebitis or emboli, varicose veins, congestive heart failure, myocardial infarction, or malignant disease, and patients who are obese or pregnant. Postoperative patients and individuals with trauma to the pelvis or lower extremities must also be considered as high risks for pulmonary embolus. These patients must be constantly assessed. Anticoagulant therapy is usually used for those patients known to be susceptible.

Recognition. The signs and symptoms of a pulmonary embolus are variable and depend on the size and location of the embolus. The clinical history and physical findings may include any one or a combination of the following: mild, transient, or marked dyspnea; mild pleural pain or persistent severe chest pain; cough; hemoptysis; tachycardia; fever; mild to severe anxiety; tachypnea or air hunger; diaphoresis; cyanosis; shock; and congestive heart failure. The physiologic effects depend on the size and number of emboli causing the pulmonary artery obstruction.

Diagnostic studies for pulmonary embolism are a chest x-ray, electrocardiogram, white blood cell count, serum enzyme and arterial blood gas determinations, radioisotope lung scan, and pulmonary angiogram.

The chest x-ray may show nonspecific findings such as an elevated diaphragm, decreased vascularity, and dilated pulmonary arteries, but frequently no abnormalities appear.

The electrocardiogram may be normal; however, a right ventricular strain pattern may be seen.

The white blood cell count may be normal or only slightly elevated. There is usually an elevation of the lactic acid dehydrogenase (LDH) but the serum glutamic-oxaloacetic transaminase (SGOT) is usually normal. The serum bilirubin may be elevated when there is right ventricular strain. Low arterial blood gas pressures (PCO_2 and PO_2) are indicative of massive pulmonary embolism.

A pulmonary angiogram is the most effective method of diagnosing pulmonary emboli. This procedure, due to its inherent complications and dangers, is performed less frequently than the radioisotope lung scan, which also may yield a definitive diagnosis.

Treatment. Nursing intervention should be directed toward treatment of shock, if present; treatment of respiratory distress; and emotional support of the patient.

The primary medical therapy is anticoagulant medication. Shock, if present, is treated with vasoconstrictors. The patient's anxiety and pain are treated with sedation. Continuous oxygen in high saturation is administered for the respiratory distress.

Surgical treatment may be necessary in any of the following situations: a contraindication to anticoagulation, recurrence of emboli during adequate anticoagulant therapy, or recurrent or near-fatal pulmonary emboli. The three surgical procedures are ligation of the vein to prevent the embolus from travelling to the heart, vena cava plication to trap the emboli, and embolectomy to remove the emboli from the pulmonary arteries.

FAT EMBOLUS. In fat embolism the primary target is the lung; therefore, fat embolism is a respiratory problem.

Two theories exist regarding the origin of embolic fat which causes the fat embolism syndrome. The first theory states that fat which originates at the site of trauma gains access to the venous circulation through small, ruptured marrow veins. This is known as the mechanical theory. The second theory is a physiochemical one which states that the alteration of lipid stability in the blood caused by the stress of trauma results in coalescence of fat particles of sufficient size to be entrapped by the lung capillaries. Regardless of whether the cause is mechanical or physiochemical, the result is twofold: the free fatty acids created by the lung's response to the fat particles are toxic to the surrounding lung substance; and alveolar collapse occurs, which not only reduces the normal oxygen diffusion but also diverts unoxygenated venous blood into the arterial circulation, thus allowing the embolic fat to reach the systemic circulation. The secondary target organs — brain, skin, eyes, and kidneys — are affected through the fat particles in the systemic circulation.

Prevention. The only known preventive measure for fat embolus is the appropriate splinting of fractures from injury to treatment.

The nurse must be cognizant of those patients who are considered at high risk for fat emboli. The incidence is usually higher with a closed fracture of a long bone, especially the femur, and the incidence increases with the number and size of the broken bones. Usually a patient with fat embolism syndrome is relatively young, with multiple fractures sustained in a vehicular accident.

Since nursing intervention cannot be directed toward preventive measures, the constant assessment of impending fat embolism syndrome must be of primary importance in the care plan.

Recognition. Classic fat embolism syndrome is characterized by a symptom-free 12- to 36-hour interval and then a rapid onset; however, it can occur as early as 3 hours or as late as 1 week after injury.

The first indication of fat embolism is the alteration of consciousness. Typically, a patient who appeared lucid and rational on admission becomes talkative and belligerent, then confused and delirious. A frank coma may ensue. Other clinical manifestations are tachypnea, tachycardia, and fever.

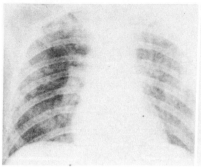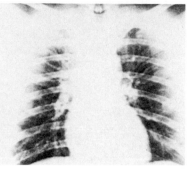

Figure 4-57. Note the snow-storm appearance of the chest x-ray on the left in a case of fat embolism.

Petechiae may be found on the conjunctiva, soft palate, axillas, and anterior part of the chest; these areas should be assessed frequently. Although the primary target is the lungs, the clinical manifestations first noted will be the effects on the secondary target organs.

The laboratory test consistently helpful in confirming the diagnosis is an arterial blood gas determination. A PO_2 of less than 60 millimeters of mercury in a patient with clinical findings indicative of fat embolus should be treated as having fat embolus. The platelet count is decreased.

The chest x-ray shows the typical so-called snow storm pulmonary filtrate (Fig. 4-57).

The electrocardiogram may show prominent S waves, arrhythmias, inversion of T waves, and right bundle branch block.

Treatment. The treatment is primarily directed toward respiratory support. Forty percent oxygen is begun by mask; however, intubation with a volume respirator or a tracheostomy may be necessary.

Pharmacologic agents including steroids, heparin, intravenous alcohol, carbohydrate infusion, and low-molecular-weight dextran are used.

Additional measures include careful control of intake and output with adequate but not excessive hydration, correction of acidosis, and replacement of any blood loss.

Decubitus Ulcers

A decubitus ulcer is an area of necrosis of the skin and underlying tissues caused by pressure (Fig. 4-58). These occur over bony prominences exposed to pressure and friction.

Prevention. Although any individual who is immobilized for an extended period of time is a candidate for the development of pressure areas, there are certain contributing factors which increase the likelihood of the occurrence of decubitus ulcers.

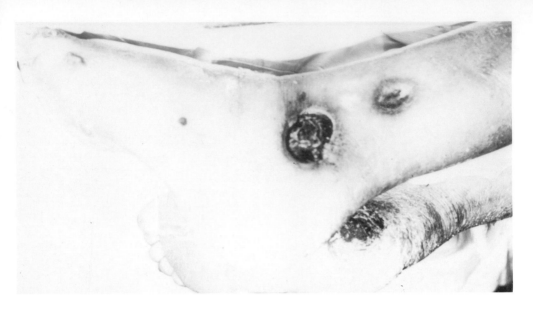

Figure 4-58. Decubiti.

These include poor nutritional state; presence of motor paralysis that causes atrophy and thus a decrease in padding over the bony prominences; loss of sensation in an area; shearing forces; edema; moisture on the area; and friction.

In the nursing care plan the nurse must provide the measures that will prevent the occurrence of decubitus ulcers. All nursing actions should be directed toward keeping the skin dry, stimulating circulation, and, most importantly, relieving or removing pressure.

Patients should be encouraged to be as active as possible. Active exercises, when possible, should be employed; if the patient is unable to carry out these exercises, passive exercises must be performed.

Patients must be turned frequently and positioned with supports such as pillows. Padding should be placed above and below bony prominences or known pressure areas, *never* directly under the suspected pressure area.

Many commercial products, such as alternating pressure mattresses, sheepskin padding and fluid-supported mattresses, are available to assist in relieving or removing pressure. The use of these should be encouraged, especially when there are anticipated pressure problems.

The nurse should also take care of the patient's hygienic and nutritional needs, remembering to inspect the skin at frequent intervals for cleanliness, dryness, and pre-pressure areas.

Patients in traction or casts must have all potential pressure areas inspected at regular intervals. Pressure from the traction apparatus or cast must be relieved immediately.

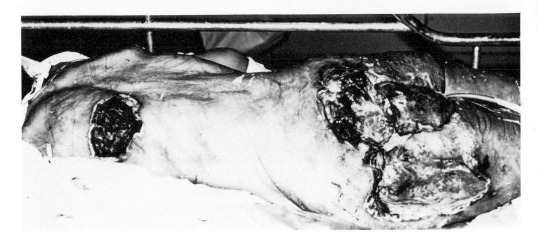

Figure 4-59. Severe pressure decubiti.

Frequently decubiti are difficult to prevent; however, their prevention is easier than the restoration of damaged skin to its normal integrity (Fig. 4-59).

Recognition. The first warning sign of a pressure area is abnormal whiteness of the skin, followed by redness and edema. The area then becomes bluish and finally black. The loss of skin occurs over this area, leaving a necrotic crater.

Treatment. The variety of treatments being used for decubitus ulcers certainly evidences the lack of a known cure. Therapy includes exposure to the air or to an ultraviolet light; application of topical agents such as granulated sugar, ointment, salt solution, mixtures of tincture of benzoin, or yeast; and the use of sprays, either plastic coating types or those containing corticosteroids and antibiotics. Regardless of the topical treatment, daily mechanical cleansing of the ulcer is necessary and continued pressure must be avoided.

All preventive measures must be continued on an even more vigorous level than usual. These should include measures for the prevention of infection.

Occasionally, surgical intervention may be necessary for débridement, closure, or grafting.

OSTEOMYELITIS. Osteomyelitis, an infection of the bone, when seen as a complication of an open fracture, surgery, or skeletal traction (by pin-tract infection) is caused by pyogenic organisms that are introduced directly through the wound. Any part of the bone may be infected, depending on the site of injury or surgery. Suppuration and necrosis occur, and the pus discharges directly through the primary wound. The infection may become chronic. The causative organism is usually *Staphylococcus,* with *Streptococcus* being less common; *Escherichia coli* and *Clostridium Welchii* are rarely involved.

Prevention. Because of the danger of infection, open fractures are treated as surgical emergencies. Initially (at the scene of the accident if possible) a sterile dressing should be laid over the wound. In the operating room, the wound is irrigated copiously with normal saline; frequently this is followed by irrigation with topical antibiotics. A débridement of nonviable tissues in the wound is also performed. The fracture is then reduced and immobilized. Generally, these patients receive large doses of antibiotics for an extended period of time.

Pins inserted for use in skeletal traction are potential sites of infection. Many orthopedic surgeons and nurses have established methods of treatment of the pin sites to prevent infection; however, there is disagreement. The most common method is covering the insertion points with sterile gauze dressing. The patient must always be informed of the necessity of leaving these areas alone. If the physician orders the cleaning of these wounds, the nurse should start at the wound and work away from it.

Patients undergoing orthopedic surgery receive preoperative scrubs of the operative and surrounding area with some type of bacteriostatic or antiseptic solution as well as a shave of the same area, which reduces the number of the microorganisms normally present on the skin. Some physicians order antibiotics to be given preoperatively. In the operating room, sterile technique is the barrier between the pyogenic organisms and the patient. Topical as well as intravenous antibiotics may be used during surgery. With the advent of total joint replacements, some hospitals have installed laminar air flow or similar systems as a further preventive measure.

Recognition. The onset of osteomyelitis is rapid. The individual feels and looks ill. Pain is usually present over the infected bone and the overlying skin is warmer than normal. The adjacent joint is often distended. The patient has an elevated temperature that either fails to return to normal or rises several days later. Examination or aspiration of the wound reveals a purulent discharge.

A blood cell count usually reveals a marked polymorphonuclear leukocytosis and an increased erthrocyte sedimentation rate.

The x-rays are negative for the first 7 to 10 days. The first finding is that of a localized area of bone destruction surrounded by an area of decalcified bone. Later the periosteal shadow is elevated. As more bone is destroyed, a motheaten appearance is seen.

A culture is made for the identification of the infecting organism and its sensitivity to antibiotics.

Treatment. When this complication is suspected, even before determination of the causative organism antibiotics are given in large doses and continued indefinitely. Antibiotics are usually begun before the identity of the organism and its sensitivity are determined.

Because the infection is contained in such a closed space, immediate drainage is a necessity. Dramatic relief is seen after drainage.

The treatment of osteomyelitis is directed not only toward the treatment of the acute initial condition, but also toward the prevention of resultant septicemia or pyemia, extension of the infection to the adjacent joint, damage to the epiphyseal cartilage in children which would cause retardation of growth, and, lastly, a state of chronic infection.

COMPARTMENT SYNDROME. Compartment syndromes are progressive vascular compromises in the forearm and leg. These are caused by swelling of the muscle (after injury or surgery) in a closed space. When this swelling occurs there is venous and arterial compression which may lead to arterial occlusion and muscle ischemia. This complication is most frequently seen following a fracture of the elbow, forearm, or tibia; crush injuries; burns; and occasionally anticoagulant therapy.

Prevention. After injury and as treatment, all extremities must be elevated higher than the heart to reduce swelling. Ice caps or packs may be applied over the affected part to reduce swelling in some cases.

Casts or other circular wraps are applied anticipating swelling of the extremity, and in some instances the cast may be bivalved at the time of treatment of the injury.

The single most important preventive measure is recognition of the signs of impending vascular compromise.

Recognition. The 5 "P's" of impending vascular compromise must be constantly evaluated when the injury is one that lends itself to this feared complication. The nurse can prevent the irreversible changes of this syndrome by constant observation and by reporting pertinent changes to the physician.

The 5 "P's" are progressive pain, pain on passive motion (when muscles are passively stretched), progressive loss of motion, paresthesias or progressive loss of sensation, and pulselessness. *Progressive pain* and *pain on passive motion* are the two most important warning signs of impending vascular compromise. Frequently the extremity is in a cast and the pulse cannot be evaluated; however, the absence of a pulse is the last sign noted before muscle ischemia occurs.

Treatment. At the first signs of vascular compromise the extremity should be further elevated. Do not continue to give medication for increasing pain. The attending physician should be notified immediately. The constrictive wraps (casts or dressings) must be released immediately; a cast should be bivalved (medially and laterally) and the circular wrapping beneath it cut. If there is no improvement, fasciotomy may be necessary.

An impending vascular compromise should always be recognized and reported by the nurse.

VOLKMANN'S ISCHEMIC CONTRACTURE. Volkmann's ischemic contracture, a flexion contracture of the wrist and fingers, is the result of ischemic necrosis of the forearm muscles in which hand function is seriously impaired. It is the end result of a flexor compartment syndrome. Volkmann described a similar condition occasionally seen in the lower extremity. This complication is preventable by following all principles outlined for the compartment syndrome. In the established stage, restoration to normal is impossible.

CONTRACTURE DEFORMITY. Contracture deformity, a permanent contracture of a joint, is caused by allowing an extremity to remain in a fixed position for long periods of time because of pain, swelling, lack of exercise, or muscle spasticity. The contracture may be due to scarring or shortening of the fibrous joint capsule or of the muscles and tendons that span the joint.

Prevention. Active or passive exercises, or both, of all joints must be encouraged in the immobilized, inactive individual. Frequent changes of position with appropriate joint support and an established exercise program must be a part of the nursing care plan. Preventable contractures should never be allowed to occur. If a joint is moved through its normal range of motion actively or passively several times daily, a contracture will not develop.

Recognition. The most common contracture deformity seen is one of flexion (especially the hip and knee), which limits the extension of the joint. Other contractures commonly seen are adduction contractures (hip and shoulder) and equinus contractures of the foot when strong plantar flexors (gastrocnemius) shorten secondary to foot drop or an unsupported foot position.

Treatment. Once a contracture is established, not only is the rehabilitation period extended but the contracture requires extensive therapy and occasionally surgery. Serial casting and traction may be helpful.

PARALYTIC ILEUS. Paralytic ileus is a frequent complication in fractures of the spine and following major surgery of the hip or back. There is absent or diminished peristalsis due to the traumatic disturbance of the autonomic nervous system; however, there is no physical obstruction or interrupted blood supply of the intestines.

Prevention. Those individuals considered to be susceptible to this complication are treated prophylactically with intravenous fluids and minimum fluids by mouth until peristalsis is established after injury or surgery. Intake by mouth is then begun slowly until no further problems with peristalsis are encountered.

Abdominal setting exercises (isometric) are encouraged within the limits of pain, as well as general bed exercises.

Recognition. Bowel sounds are diminished or absent. This may be the only clinical manifestation in the early stages. Abdominal distension is usually prominent and the abdomen is tense. Constipation is present and small amounts of flatus may or may not be passed. Vomiting occurs after eating. The pain is usually dull and diffuse.

Treatment. The physician should be notified of a suspected paralytic ileus immediately.

The gastrointestinal tract is rested by allowing nothing by mouth and maintaining fluid balance through intravenous fluids. A rectal tube may help to reduce distension. A naso gastric tube may be inserted and connected to suction in the more serious cases.

This complication is usually resolved within 72 hours after surgery or injury.

POSTOPERATIVE DISLOCATION. Postoperative dislocation may occur after surgery for insertion of a femoral head prosthesis or a total hip replacement (femoral head and acetabular components). In either case, the artificial head dislocates from the acetabulum. This can occur with incorrect positional changes due to the surgical break in the integrity of the hip joint, since the capsule and the muscle surrounding the hip joint have been surgically incised. The dislocation may occur posteriorly or anteriorly.

Prevention. Following surgery for insertion of a femoral head prosthesis or a total hip replacement, the involved extremity should be placed in a position of abduction with 0 to 15 degrees of external rotation.

Positions of adduction or acute flexion and extremes of rotation must be avoided at all times.

Abduction may be maintained by use of an abduction splint, Buck's or split Russell's traction, or simply by placing two pillows between the legs.

These basic principles must be applied when turning the patient: never let the leg drop into adduction, acutely flex, or assume a position of extreme rotation. Generally, two persons are needed to turn a patient after hip surgery.

Recognition. Following dislocation, the patient experiences severe pain and can usually determine that the hip is out of place.

The extremity assumes a position of external rotation, adduction, and shortening with an anterior dislocation, and a position of internal rotation and adduction with a posterior dislocation.

Treatment. The physician should be notified immediately and the patient made as comfortable as possible until his or her arrival. No attempt should be made to reduce the hip.

The physician usually reduces the hip using analgesics; however, it may be necessary to place the patient under general anesthesia in order to accomplish this. Only rarely is an open reduction required.

Following reduction, the patient is treated as initially postoperatively concerning hip management.

PERONEAL NERVE PALSY. Peroneal nerve palsy is a partial or complete paralysis of the peroneal nerve due to any cause. It is most commonly seen in elderly patients with very little normal subcutaneous padding, who lie with an injured lower extremity in external rotation so that pressure occurs over the peroneal nerve just as it crosses forward beneath the neck of the fibula (Fig. 4-60). It also can occur when pressure is present in this same area from traction wrapping or from a cast (Fig. 4-61). Injury to the nerve causes weakness or paralysis of the dorsiflexors of the foot.

Prevention. Prevention of peroneal nerve palsy lies in prevention of pressure over the peroneal nerve. The injured extremity should be supported on a pillow which is fluffed up so that there is no pressure over the lateral side of the knee as the leg lies in external rotation. If traction is applied, the traction straps should extend above the end of the fibula or else stop sufficiently below the nerve so that pressure from neither the traction strap nor the elastic bandage wrapping occurs at the peroneal nerve site. A cast has to be similarly padded so that no pressure occurs over the neck of the fibula.

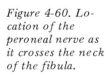

Figure 4-60. Location of the peroneal nerve as it crosses the neck of the fibula.

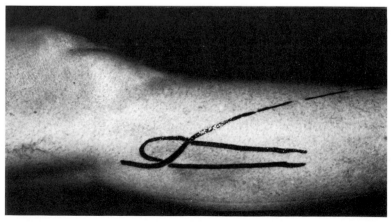

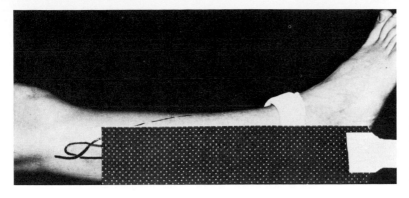

Figure 4-61. Do not allow straps or elastic wrap to cause pressure over the peroneal nerve.

Recognition. Inability to strongly dorsiflex the foot, combined with numbness or paresthesia over the dorsolateral aspect of the foot, is the clinical sign of peroneal nerve pressure. If the nerve is further traumatized there may be complete paralysis of the muscles of the anterior compartment so that the patient cannot actively dorsiflex the foot; this may result in foot drop.

Treatment. After a peroneal nerve palsy has occurred, the treatment consists of prevention of contracture by passive dorsiflexion exercises of the foot and ankle several times daily, appropriate support, and positioning the foot so that it does not lie in an equinus position. A dorsiflexion brace may also be needed when the patient walks while the peroneal nerve is recovering from injury. Fortunately, spontaneous recovery usually occurs.

TRAUMATIC NEURITIS. Traumatic neuritis of the ulnar nerve may occur in the bedridden patient who uses the elbows to push up in bed. This may irritate the ulnar nerve as it passes subcutaneously around the medial epicondyle of the elbow.

Prevention. The patient must be taught to use the overhead trapeze and to avoid elbow pressure. The elbows should be padded.

Recognition. The clinical picture is manifested by numbness and discomfort in the ulnar nerve distribution to the hand with tingling and numbness in the ring and little fingers. A complete palsy may occur with paralysis of the muscles in the hand innervated by the ulnar nerve.

RELATED SYSTEMS. Obviously any patient who has been subjected to trauma, surgery, or a serious illness has an increased likelihood of complications of related systems — circulatory, respiratory, gastrointestinal, and genitourinary — which have not been discussed here. These are covered in many texts and the reader is directed to review those known or predicted conditions occurring in any immobilized patient.

WEDGE STRYKER FRAME. The wedge Stryker frame (or a similar turning device) is essential in many different nursing problems, such as severe multiple injuries, quadriplegia and paraplegia, severe decubitus ulcers, severe burns, head injuries, and cervical spinal injuries. It is, however, contraindicated in extremely obese, comatose, disoriented, or restless patients, and in young children.

Frequent changes in position, which the frame allows, aid in increasing circulation, which improves tissue nourishment, thereby promoting healing and preventing tissue edema.

Skeletal cervical traction can be used easily with the frame. Countertraction can be accomplished by placing the frame in a reverse Trendelenburg position.

Personnel caring for a patient on the frame must be familiar with its parts. The two main parts are the posterior frame, which is used when the patient is lying on his back, and the anterior frame, which is used when the patient is lying on his abdomen. The anterior frame has a face mask which supports the forehead but allows the mouth and nose to be unobstructed. Other parts of the frame include an elevation lock, which enables the bed to be elevated to the Trendelenburg position; a circle lock, which, when depressed, unlocks and opens the circle; a turning lock, which controls turning; a stop button, which stops the rotation of the frame when the lower frame is level and the lock pin is over the locking hole; a nylon stop lock, which stops the frame when the rotation is complete; and a caster guide, which prevents sideways movement but allows longitudinal movement.

Canvas covers are applied to the frame in the following manner. They are arranged on the posterior frame in three sections: the first section is from the top of the frame to the symphysis pubis, the second section is for the perineal area, and the third section is from the perineal area to the ankles. The anterior frame has a molded face piece; the canvas covers on this frame begin at the shoulders and extend to the symphysis pubis, with a separate section for the perineal area and the last canvas cover extending from the perineal area to the ankles.

Linens are applied over the canvas covers. They may consist of special linens with ties or sheets folded to fit the sections and pinned into place. Linens should be changed at least every 24 hours, or more frequently if they become soiled. Linens should always be free of wrinkles.

Being turned on the frame is a frightening experience for the patient. A thorough explanation must be given to the patient before the turning procedure begins; he or she should be told that it is neither dangerous nor painful.

Although the frame is designed so that one person can turn

it without difficulty, having two persons available not only instills confidence in the patient, but offers reassurance to the operator of the frame as well. Application of two restraining straps around the frame also reassures the patient.

The wheels of the frame are locked and all extra equipment, such as pillows, the call light and tubing, is removed. The anterior or posterior frame is placed over the patient and secured in place. Releasing the turning lock allows the frame to be turned.

Clothing tends to wrinkle, causing discomfort and potential pressure areas; therefore, it is usually not used when a patient is on a frame. Privacy should be ensured by the use of sheets.

A bedpan can be placed under the patient by removing the perineal section, placing the bedpan on a strap or rack, and raising it up under the patient. The bedpan should not be left under the patient continuously because this position allows the buttocks to sag through the frame.

A footboard is placed on the frame when the patient is on his back to prevent foot drop.

Before caring for a patient in a Stryker frame, all personnel should familiarize themselves with the parts of the frame and the actual turning procedure. The literature which accompanies the frame must be available at all times to personnel using the frame.

Whether the patient is lying supine or prone, good body alignment and support must always be maintained. Small pillows or other padding should be used, just as with a patient on a regular bed. Marked deformities of the hips or knees may require the use of pillows; these must be placed in the appropriate positions before the turning procedure is carried out.

Prism glasses can benefit the patient in the supine position by enlarging his visual field.

The turning routine will depend on the diagnosis, but the patient is usually turned every 2 hours. All skin should be inspected immediately following the turning procedure.

CIRCOLECTRIC BED. The CircOlectric bed (Fig. 4-62) is used for the same nursing problems as the wedge Stryker frame. In addition, it may be used for any patient who requires frequent changes of position or when problems with ambulation are anticipated. It is not effectively used with patients for whom the prone position is contraindicated.

This bed allows the nurse to turn a patient from the supine to the prone position and to place him or her in any position from the Trendelenburg to erect stance. Thus, many of the hazards of immobility are prevented.

Almost every type of traction, including cervical skeletal traction, can be maintained on this bed.

Turning is accomplished by an electric control device which fits in the operator's hand.

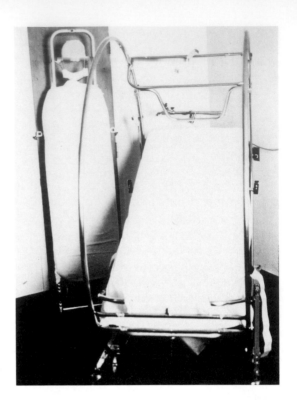

Figure 4-62. Circ-Olectric bed.

The bed consists of a 360-degree frame, anterior and posterior mattresses, linens, armboards, restraining straps, additional springs which may be added under the mattress for obese patients, and optional equipment which includes traction bars, pulleys, an accessories basket, and transfer slings.

The turning procedure is similar to that for the Stryker frame. The anterior or posterior frame is secured in place; restraining straps are placed around the buttocks and breast line; and the control button is pressed. The straps are then removed, the head stud nut is unscrewed, and the top frame is raised and attached to the safety bar. In case of a mechanical failure, a hand crank is used to complete the turning procedure.

The literature which accompanies the bed must be available at all times to the personnel using the bed. All personnel should familiarize themselves with it before caring for a patient on the bed.

The turning routine as well as the variety of allowed positions will depend on the patient's condition.

All nursing measures are the same as for the patient on the Stryker frame.

The CircOlectric bed allows the patient to gradually assume the stance position for ambulation and is frequently used for

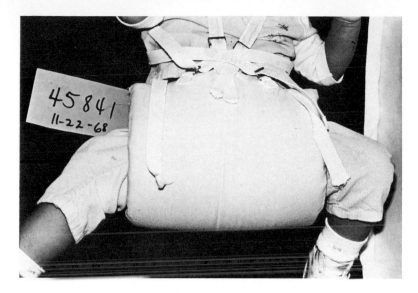

Figure 4-63.
Frejka abduction
splint.

this purpose. The patient is brought to the standing position and walks off the bed.

BRACES. Braces are used to maintain certain positions, to allow better function, as supportive measures, and to prevent certain movements. The variety of braces is almost endless. Although there are some standard braces, they are usually individually designed for each patient.

Abduction braces and splints are of varied design. Regardless of the type, they are all used to maintain the hip or hips in an abducted position (Fig. 4-63).

If a brace is to be worn, the patient must be instructed in its application and care. The brace should be kept clean (leather soap can be used as needed); it should be allowed to aerate when not being worn; nothing should be allowed to rest on the brace when it is not being worn; and the joints should be oiled frequently. Corrections should not be made on the brace without consulting the physician or orthotist.

The patient should report to the physician or orthotist any noisy joints or poor alignment; excessive motion in joints from wear; worn or broken straps and cuffs; rust; broken or missing parts; irritation or rashes of any skin areas resulting from pressure; and excessive wear of heels and soles of the shoe if it is part of the brace. Discomfort or pain caused by the brace should also be reported.

Activity allowed in the brace will be directed by the physician.

The most common braces with which the orthopedic nurse should be familiar are as follows:

Klenzak short leg dorsiflexion brace — used to substitute dynamically for absent or weak dorsiflexors; corrects a drop foot and lifts the foot into dorsiflexion.

Short leg dorsiflexion spring brace — used to assist weak dorsiflexors and prevent drop foot (Fig. 4-64).

Short leg double upright brace with posterior strap — prevents drop foot by limiting plantar flexion of the foot in the brace at neutral position.

Long leg double upright brace with drop-lock knee — used to stabilize the paralyzed, weak, unstable, or arthritic knee. When necessary, the lock is dropped into position to keep the knee from flexing.

Cock-up dorsiflexion wrist brace — used to maintain the painful, arthritic, or weakened wrist in the dorsiflexed position of function.

Abduction (airplane splint) shoulder brace — used to support the shoulder in a position of abduction after rotator cuff surgery.

Back brace — grips the pelvis and chest to limit motion of the spine. Many styles and designs are utilized.

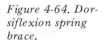

Figure 4-64. Dorsiflexion spring brace.

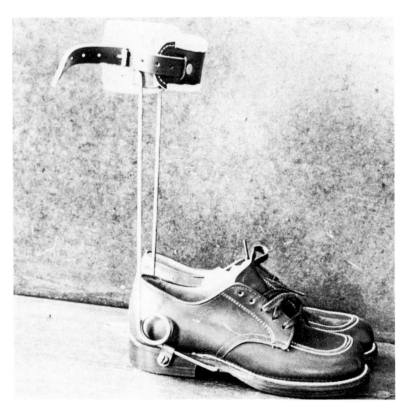

SOFT GOODS MATERIALS. A tremendous number of soft goods materials are used for protection and support. These include rib belts; a variety of arm, hand, finger, ankle, and knee splints; cervical collars; clavicle straps; lumbosacral corsets; arm slings; and arm immobilizers.

One should become familiar with the soft goods used in a specific institution. Practice in applying these devices to herself or to another member of the staff helps the nurse to become confident in using them.

Rehabilitation

Ideally, the physician, the nurse, and the family work together in the proper education of the patient so that the desired activity or physical therapy program is explained to and performed by the patient. It is important to remember that the exercises are to be performed and the modalities of treatment applied regardless of who supervises the patient.

The nurse should have a basic understanding of all of the many areas involved in physical therapy. Much of the patient's education comes from the direct supervision of the nurse, as certainly do most of his or her daily activities.

TERMINOLOGY OF RANGE OF MOTION EXERCISES. Range of motion is often abbreviated as ROM. This is the number of degrees through which a joint moves.

Progressive resistance exercise is often abbreviated as PRE. The strength of the muscle is increased by exercising it against increasing resistance. This is usually done very gradually.

Setting or isometric exercise refers to tensing of the muscle or muscles and making them firm. The muscle length does not change. Such exercises are usually done slowly to the count of three. The patient simply sets or makes a muscle hard, and does not attempt to move the body, limb, or joint through any particular motion. This is a way of improving muscle tone without moving the joint or trunk where the muscle attaches.

Active exercises are being done when the patient uses his or her own muscles to do the exercises.

Passive exercise is being performed when the patient does not use his or her own muscles; some person or assistive device must do the exercise.

Range of motion exercises should be done for every joint at least 10 times a day for the immobilized patient. Range of motion exercises for affected or injured joints will depend on the physician's instructions.

GENERAL BED EXERCISES. General bed exercises are an integral part of overall patient care on most orthopedic services. Most patients, regardless of their orthopedic problem, can participate in general bed exercises, with certain limitations depending on their particular difficulty.

The advantages for a patient who does general bed exercises are maintenance and improvement of muscle tone and function; prevention of skin problems, improvement in general body and tissue circulation; improvement in respiratory, cardiac, gastrointestinal, and genitourinary function; and, last but not least, allowing the patient to participate in his own care.

The general bed exercises are as follows: With the patient lying on his back and straight in bed, teach him to straighten the knees and to try to touch the foot of the bed with the toes, at the same time alternating flexion and extension of the foot. The muscles should be held hard while doing this. Instruct the patient to gradually stretch his legs toward the foot of the bed or wall and at the same time keep the knees straight. This exercise will tighten up the quadriceps, the muscles on top of the thigh. When the patient dorsiflexes and plantar flexes the foot he is exercising the muscles of the calf and foreleg. He should be instructed to straighten the knees, push the legs down against the bed and tighten the buttocks muscles. When the patient straightens the knees, the quadriceps (anterior thigh muscles) are brought into action. Thus, when he pushes the legs down against the bed he brings the gluteus maximus (buttocks muscle) into action. This may sometimes be better understood by the patient if you tell him to push his heels against the bed. He should hold this position steadily and firmly for a slow count of three. After that he is to rest for a few seconds, as completely relaxed as possible, and then repeat the exercise.

With the hands on the abdomen, the patient should raise the neck and shoulders far enough to tighten the stomach muscles. Depending on the patient's age and general musculature, this exercise can be made more vigorous by having him lift the head and shoulders even farther. Also, if there is some back problem or if no actual flexion of the spine is desired, this exercise can be done by having the patient lift the head and neck only off the pillow, just enough to tighten the stomach and abdomen muscles but without any back motion.

Stretching the arms overhead, the patient takes a deep breath and tries to touch the head of the bed or wall behind the bed. This increases respiratory function and also exercises the muscles that elevate and rotate the shoulders.

With his arms at his sides, the patient presses the shoulders and head against the bed, trying to pinch the shoulder blades together. This exercise tightens the muscles of the back and posterior shoulder region. It also tightens and strengthens the posterior neck muscles.

These exercises are done at least four times daily, repeating each exercise five to twenty times. Frequency and duration of general bed exercises are tailored to the individual's general condition.

TRANSFER ACTIVITIES. Transfer activities consist of moving the patient from bed to chair, bed to commode, and bed to wheelchair. During this activity the patient should be encouraged to use all unaffected extremities, helping himself as much as possible. First the patient should be moved toward the edge of the bed and assisted to a sitting position by having the patient push up on his elbows while you lift his shoulders with one arm and swing his legs over the edge of the bed with the other arm. He is then assisted to the standing position, making sure his feet are firmly planted on the floor, face the patient and firmly grasp each side of the rib cage while pushing your knee against one of his knees. This tends to lock the knee into full extension as the patient comes to a standing position. Once the patient is in the full upright position, have him pivot on his good leg, positioning him to sit in the chair. The patient may walk to his affected or unaffected side, depending on his preference; however, most medical personnel ambulate patients to the unaffected side.

Even though the patient may not be allowed to bear weight on the extremity, it is safer for him to place his foot on the floor to rest rather than to hold it above the floor.

CRUTCH WALKING. There are many different types of crutches. The most common types are the wooden, so-called axillary crutches, which have handles for the hands and a top axillary portion which goes under the arms. There are other types of crutches which are applicable in certain instances; for example, Lofstrand crutches which hook onto the arms just above the elbows, and platform crutches which are a modification of axillary crutches. If an individual cannot straighten out his elbows and wishes to put his weight on the bent elbow rather than on the hands and wrists, platform crutches are utilized. The body weight is transmitted to the floor through the trunk, arms, and crutches, rather than through the lower extremity. The lower extremity can be spared weight bearing wholly or in part depending on how the crutches are used.

By far the most common gait pattern used on crutches in orthopedics is the so-called three-point gait. Three-point gait means that as weight is borne on the affected lower extremity, for instance the left, there are three points on the floor, in this case both crutches and the left leg (Fig. 4-65). If three-point non-weight bearing is desired, the third point (the leg) is not to touch the floor at all. Three-point gait is utilized when the hip or leg on only one side of the body needs protection.

A four-point gait is used when both lower extremities — for

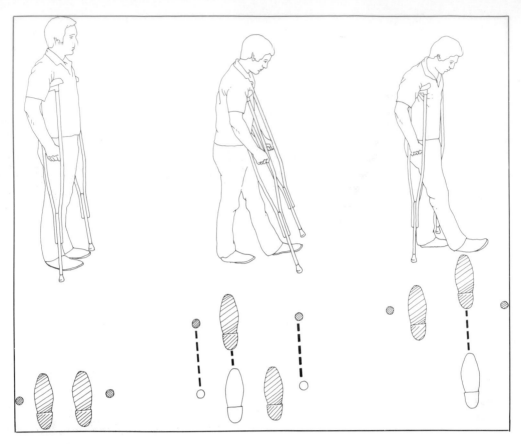

Figure 4-65.
Three-point gait.

example, in bilateral arthritis of the hip — need partial protection. Three points are on the floor at all times. The sequence is: right crutch, left foot, left crutch, right foot (Fig. 4-66). This is a slow but stable gait and the patient's weight is constantly being shifted.

In a two-point gait there are two points in contact with the floor at all times. The right crutch and the left foot go forward together and then the left crutch and the right foot follow (Fig. 4-67). Patients on a four-point gait move to this two-point gait as strength improves and the need for protection decreases.

The swing-through gait is one in which both crutches are moved forward and then the body weight is lifted and swung to meet the crutches; or, the crutches may be moved forward and the body lifted and swung beyond them (Fig. 4-68).

In preparation for use of crutches, the patient's upper musculature should be strengthened as well as other muscles which are needed for ambulation, such as the quadriceps, gluteals, and hip abductors.

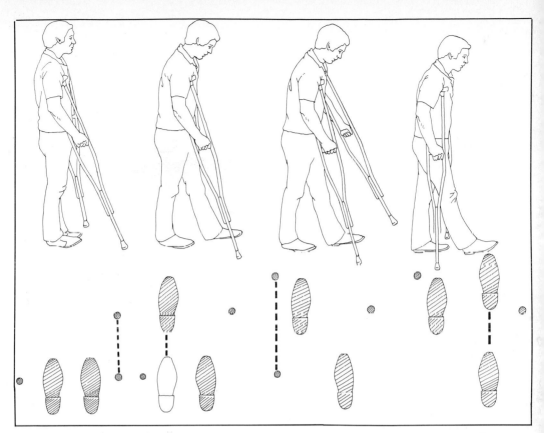

Figure 4-66. Four-point gait.

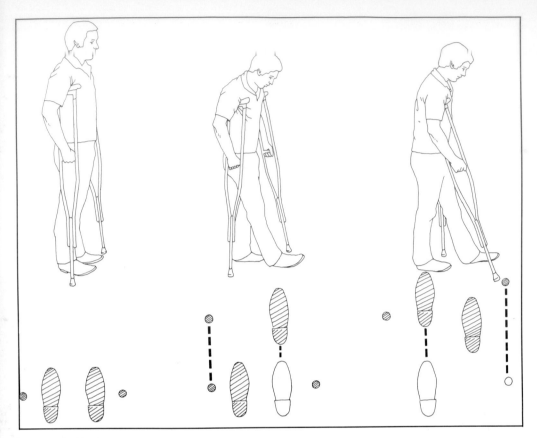

Figure 4-67. Two-point gait.

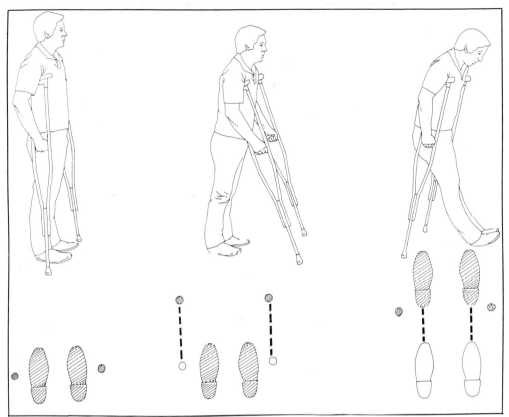

Figure 4-68.
Swing-through
gait.

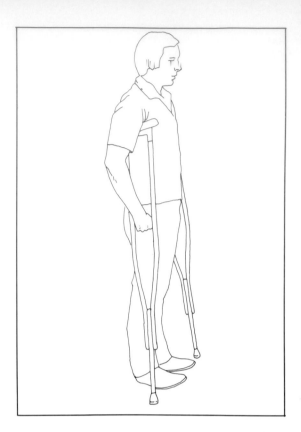

Figure 4-69. Appropriate adjustment of crutches.

The patient must be appropriately fitted for crutches. They should be an inch or an inch and a half from the armpits, and with the patient standing the elbows should be flexed 30 degrees (Fig. 4-69). Large rubber suction-tips should be placed on the ends of the crutches so that they will not slide. The patient should be instructed not to bear weight on the axillary portion of the crutch but to bear the weight on his hands. This promotes good balance and posture and prevents damage to the radial nerve by axillary pressure (so-called crutch palsy).

When instructing a patient in the use of crutches, he should always be shown how to use this support as well as the expected gait. Never hand a patient a pair of crutches, verbally instruct him in the appropriate gait, and expect him to be able to accomplish it.

When it is necessary for the individual using crutches to go up and down stairs, it is important that he be taught the appropriate method for this. The patient should be instructed as follows: stop at the bottom of the stairs, and if the bannister is on the right, shift the crutches to the left hand; then take the bannister with the right hand, place the stronger leg on the first stair, and, pushing on the crutches in the left hand and pulling on the bannister with the right hand, bring the involved extremity up onto the stair with the stronger extremity. The crutches are then brought up on the stair also, and the process is repeated stair by stair. When descending, just the reverse is done: crutches are shifted to the right hand and the railing is grasped in the left hand. The crutches go down first; then the weaker, involved leg is placed on the down step with the crutches, using the crutches and the bannister; and the stronger leg is brought down last. The basic rule of stairs is: strong leg up first and down last.

USE OF A WALKER. A walker is used in lieu of crutches when it is felt that it will be safer and easier for the patient. This is commonly the case in elderly patients who lack stamina and dexterity.

There are different types of walkers. In general, the light-weight pick-up walker requires less exertion and is probably more widely used than any other.

The patient is instructed to grasp the walker firmly and comfortably, to advance it slightly in front, and then to step forward in the pattern that feels normal. One can teach the individual a three-point type of gait in which the walker represents two points and the involved extremity, the third point. It is also used in the same manner for non-weight bearing, in which case the foot is only allowed to rest on the floor rather than to bear weight. The patient may progress from a walker to crutches when he or she develops the strength and ability to handle crutches safely.

USE OF A CANE. A cane is used on the side opposite the involved extremity. The body weight is then maintained by the cane and the weak extremity while the uninvolved limb is moved forward (Fig. 4-70). The cane must have a rubber suction-tip and should allow a comfortable grip. The patient's elbow should be allowed to flex 25 to 30 degrees when the cane is the proper length. There are adjustable aluminum canes available as well as wooden ones. A cane primarily aids in balance and in relieving compression forces working on the hip joint. Ordinarily, when bearing weight in the stance phase, a force of approximately 2.5 times body weight is exerted across the hip joint to keep the pelvis from dropping. A small amount of pressure on a cane in the opposite hand (long lever arm) can act equal and opposite to the weight of the body's center of gravity working on a short lever arm; thereby the pelvis will not drop and the abductor force is not needed to stabilize the pelvis. The hip joint is spared this entire pressure with each step, thereby becoming more comfortable.

PATIENT AND FAMILY EDUCATION. A knowledgeable pa-

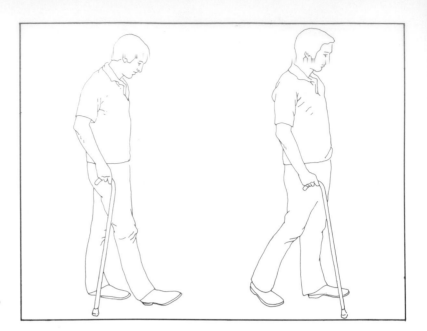

Figure 4-70. Use of a cane; left hip involved.

tient is a much more cooperative patient. The orthopedic nurse must begin to educate the patient and family when the patient is first seen on admission, in the emergency room, or in the clinic.

The patient and others who will be involved in his care can only participate in the setting of realistic goals from a base of knowledge.

The individual must be aware that he is the primary instrument of his own rehabilitation, and he must know that the length of the recovery period is often directly proportional to his involvement. However, it is the orthopedic nurse's responsibility to supply the patient with a simple explanation of his condition and the necessary skills to obtain maximum return of function consistent with his condition or with the disease process, injury, or surgery.

Patients under stress tend to forget verbal explanations; therefore, written materials describing expected performances should be given to him. The use of sound-slides and videotapes is helpful in reinforcing the verbal and written information. Patients must not be expected to remember lengthy explanations or the specific steps of an unfamiliar procedure.

What is taught to the patient must be as carefully planned as the other aspects of nursing care. The basic information necessary for an effective treatment program must be shared with the patient and those who will be helping him. This basic information should include cause, mechanism, treatment, and prognosis.

Teaching materials can be collected from numerous sources. Many orthopedic companies have educational materials available on request either from their representatives in the area or from the home office. When they are not available, these materials can be created.

Discharge Planning

Discharge planning is begun at the time of the patient's admission to the hopsital. The anticipated date of discharge to the home, extended care facility, or nursing home is usually known at this time.

If the patient is to return to a home setting, it is the responsibility of the nurse to assure not only the readiness of the patient for discharge but also the readiness of the family and home environment.

The status of the patient's activities of daily living must be established. Whether the patient may be independent, will need assistance, or should be supervised while doing these activities should be understood by both the patient and his or her family.

Any special equipment needed in the home should be obtained prior to discharge. This equipment might include an elevated commode seat, self-help aids, a special hospital bed, and an assistive gait device, if necessary for ambulation.

If home visits by registered nurses or other home-care personnel are needed, this must be arranged for prior to discharge. Whoever is to be home with the patient should be instructed in any necessary or appropriate care, exercises, and ambulation.

If immobilization is to be continued at home it will be necessary to instruct those persons involved in the patient's care in the appropriate positioning and skin care.

Transfers from bed to toilet, tub, shower, car, and other areas should be taught to the patient as well as to those persons who will be involved in home care.

If the patient needs an assistive gait device, such as a walker, crutches or cane, he or she and those persons involved in home care should demonstrate a knowledge of techniques for mobility on stairs with and without a rail, inclines, and street curbs. The approach to the home should be considered prior to the patient's transportation arrangements. Factors to be considered are the driveway or sidewalk space available to enter and exit from the car, steps, and the availability of a hand rail; any obstacles may necessitate transportation home in an ambulance.

If the patient is to use crutches, a walker, or a cane at home, the following suggestions are helpful in aiding safety and convenience. Throw rugs should be removed in areas where the patient will be walking, to prevent slipping and falling; furniture should be arranged so that there is plenty of room for moving about; and when doorways are not wide enough for the patient to go through straight, he or she should be taught how to turn sideways (assistance may be needed for this). If there are children in the home, toys should be kept out of the way to prevent tripping and falling, and house pets should be kept in another room or held by someone when the patient is up. If it is necessary for the patient to go up and down steps, this should be done with the assistance of a handrail or another person. The rooms should be arranged so that items which are frequently needed are convenient, and the telephone should be located where it is easily reached.

If the patient is to be alone at home most of the time, he or she should be encouraged to arrange visits from family and friends during those times when they would be most helpful, such as at bath time and meals, and during outside walking.

In general, patients and their families should be instructed to space the activity of the patient at intervals so that he or she does not become overly tired. Short, frequent walks should be taken several times daily rather than only a few long, extended ones.

Specific instructions for the post-hospital care of specific conditions or surgery which has been performed should be given to the patient *in writing*. These instructions should include skin care, activity, necessary transportation to the physician's office, clothing, special equipment needed, whether or not shower or tub baths are permissible, any special precautions, and signs and symptoms to be reported to the physician. The patient should always be supplied with the telephone number of the physician in case any problems should arise.

These discharge instructions should be developed by the nursing staff and made available to the patient prior to discharge from the hospital.

If the patient is to be transferred to an extended care facility or a nursing home, the appropriate transfer forms and orders must be provided. The level of present activity as well as anticipated functional return must also be clearly indicated.

SUGGESTED READINGS

Ackerman, Susan: The GSB total elbow. *Orthop. Nurs. Assoc. J.* 1:112–114, December 1974.

Ackerman, Susan: Silicone rubber implant, arthroplasty for the great toe. *Orthop. Nurs. Assoc. J.* 2:115, 135–137, June 1975.

Ackerman, Susan: Some new drugs and new treatments with drugs in orthopedics. *Orthop. Nurs. Assoc. J.* 2:246–247, October 1975.

Anderson, Merlin G.: Orthopedic traction and nursing care. *Orthop. Nurs. Assoc. J.* 2:304–307, December 1975.

Anonymous: How to negotiate the ups and downs, ins and outs of body alignment. *Nursing '74*, pp. 46–51, October 1974.

Apple, David F., Jr., and Jones, Irene: Neurovascular checks — what and why? *Orthop. Nurs. Assoc. J.* 1:19–21, August 1974.

Aufranc, Otto, E., and Turner, Roderick H.: Total replacement of the arthritic hip. *Hosp. Pract.*, 6:66–81, October 1971.

Bailey, Joseph A. II: Tractions, suspensions, and a ringless splint. *Am. J. Nurs.* 70:1724–1726, 1970.

Bame, Kathleen: Halo traction. *Am. J. Nurs.* 69:1933–1937, 1969.

Barki, K.: Traction and suspension ringless splint. *Am. J. Nurs.* 70:172, 1970.

Bennage, Barbara A., and Cummings, Marjorie: Nursing the patient undergoing total hip arthroplasty, *Nurs. Clin. North Am.* 8:107–116, 1973.

Beaumont, Estell: Wheelchairs. *Nursing '73*, pp. 48–57, November 1973

Blazevich, Dianne, and Weinheimer, Pati Guidelines for cast care. *Orthop. Nurs. Assoc. J.* 2:138–139, June 1975.

Blount, Walter P.: The non-operative management of scoliosis. *Orthop. Nurs. Assoc. J.* 3:19–21, January 1976.

Bradley, D.: Fractures of the pelvis. *Nurs. Times* 68:376–379, 1972.

Bradley, D.: Checking a plaster — how and why. *Nurs. Times* 70:1190–1192, 1974.

Brooks, Helen: Cotrel or red rope traction. *Orthop. Nurs. Assoc. J.* 2:173–174, July 1975.

Brower, Phyllis, et al.: Maintaining muscle function in patients on bedrest. *Am. J. Nurs.* 72:1250–1253, 1972.

Brown, Sandy: Solving the complexities of orthopedic nursing; easing the burden of traction and cast. Part I. *R.N.* 38:35–41, February 1975.

Brown, Sandy: Orthopedic nursing action. *Orthop. Nurs. Assoc. J.* 2:279–281, November 1975.

Brunner, N.A.: *Orthopedic Nursing: A Programmed Approach.* St. Louis: Mosby, 1970.

Campbell, W.C.: *Operative Orthopaedics* (5th ed.). Edited by A.H. Crenshaw. St. Louis: Mosby, 1971.

Ciuca, Rudy; Bradish, Jennie; and Trombly, Suzanne: Range of motion exercises, active and passive: A handbook. *Nursing '73*, pp. 25–37, October 1973.

Cooper, Sandra: Low back pain caused by rupturing of the nucleus pulposus. *Orthop. Nurs. Assoc. J.*, 2:224–230, September 1975.

Day, B.H.: *Orthopaedic Appliances.* London: Faber and Faber, 1972.

del Bueno, Dorothy J.: Recognizing fat embolism in patients with multiple injuries. *R.N.* 36:48–51, January 1973.

Dimon, Joseph II., and Donahoo, Clara A.: Nursing care of the patient in traction. *J. Pract. Nurs.* 22:18–19, September 1972.

Dimon, Joseph H., and Donahoo, Clara A.: Orthopedic teaching aids. *Orthop. Nurs. Assoc. J.* 2:217–219, September 1975.

Donn, Mary C.: Right total hip replacement. *Nurs. Times.* 70: 1654–1657, 1974.

Dunn, Barbara H.: Scoliosis detection. *Orthop. Nurs. Assoc. J.* 2:282–283, November 1975.

Evarts, Charles M. [ed.]: Symposium on surgery of the hip and knee. *Orthop. Clin. North Am.* 1:3–299, 1971.

Farrell, Jane: Preparing a patient for cast life. *Orthop. Nurs. Assoc. J.* 1:70–73, October 1974.

Feyock, Joanne M. Webber: A do-it-yourself restraint that works. *Nursing '75*, p. 18, January 1975.

Flaherty, P.T.: *Braces: A Primer for Nurses.* Minneapolis: American Rehabilitation Foundation, 1968.

Flemming, J.J.: Fat embolism. *Nurs. Mirror* 133:21–23, November 1971.

Foss, Georgia: Use your head and save your back — body mechanics. *Nursing '73*, pp. 25–32, May 1973.

Foss, Georgia: Breaking the architectural barrier with crutches, wheelchairs, and walkers. *Nursing '73*, pp. 16–31, October 1973.

Fowler, Marsha D.: Behold the great right toe. *Am. J. Nurs.* 74:1817–1819, 1974.

Friedmann, Lawrence W.: The quality of hope for the amputee. *Arch. Surg.* 110:760, 1975.

Glancy, Gerard L.: Compartment syndromes. *Orthop. Nurs. Assoc. J.* 2:148–151, June 1975.

Gossling, Harry R., et al: Fat embolism. *J. Bone Joint Surg.* 56[Am]: 1327–1362, 1974.

Guy, F.M.: Implants used in orthopedic surgery. Part 2 *Nurs. Times* 68:500–503, 1972.

Hadley, Richard, et al.: Adult respiratory distress syndrome without roentgenographic changes. *J. Bone Joint Surg.* 56[Am]: 396–400, 1974.

Harding, Joan M.: Amputations of the lower limb. *Nurs. Times* 70:1025–1027, 1974.

Harrold, A. J.: Laminectomy for disc disorders. *Nurs. Times* 67:406–408, 1971.

Hinsch, Lorraine A.: Nursing care of hip surgery patients. *A.O.R.N. J.,* 18:550–555, 1973.

Hitch, Melanie: Perivascular ulcerations. *Orthop. Nurs. Assoc. J.,* 2:37, February 1975.

Hodge, Bobbie, et al.: Scoliosis: Affectionate, yet firm, postoperative care. Nursing Grand Rounds. *Nursing '74*, pp. 49–55, August 1974.

Hogberg, Anne, and Tweet, Barbara: Nailing of femoral neck fractures. *Orthop. Nurs. Assoc. J.* 1:40–41, September 1974.

Hogberg, Anne: Orthopedic nursing: Preventing orthopedic complications. Part 2. *R.N.* 38:34–37, March 1975.

Hohf, Robert P., et al.: The threat of thrombophlebitis, Nursing Grand Rounds. *Nursing '73*, pp. 38–44, November 1973.

Hrobsky, Arthur: The patient on a CircOlectric bed. *Am. J. Nurs.* 71:2352–2353, 1971.

Hrobsky, Arthur: Small world of the traction patient — reducing the hazards of immobility. *Bedside Nurse* 4:27–30, December 1971.

Isler, Charlotte: Decubitus/old truths and some new ideas. *R.N.* 35:42–45, July 1972.

Johnson, Colleen F., and Convery, F. Richard: Preventing emboli after total hip replacement. *Am. J. Nurs.* 75:804–806, 1975.

Jones, V., and Killian, M.: Pulmonary embolism. *Orthop. Nurs. Assoc. J.* 2:170–172, July 1975.

Jordan, H.S., and Kavchak, M.A.: Transfer techniques. *Nursing '73*, pp. 19–22, March 1973.

Jordan, Helen, and Cypres, Robert M.: All around care for the leg amputee. *Nursing '74*, pp. 51–55, April 1974.

Kamenetz, Herman L.: Selecting a wheelchair. *Am. J. Nurs.* 72:100–101, 1972.

Kettelkamp, Donald B., and Leach, Robert [eds.]: Symposium: Total Knee Replacement. *Clin. Orthop.* 94, July-August 1973.

Killian, Marguerite A.: Continuous closed tube irrigation and suction therapy. *Orthop. Nurs. Assoc. J.* 3:16–18, January 1976.

Kurth, J.S.: Correct application of the Thomas splint and Pearson attachment. *Nursing '73*, pp. 20–24, July 1973.

Larson, Carroll B., et al.: *Orthopedic Nursing* (8th ed.). St. Louis: Mosby, 1974.

Lathrop, J.: Traction treatment. *Nursing '74*, pp. 72–73, May 1974.

Law, J.: The fat embolism syndrome. *Nurs. Clin. North Am.* 8:191–198, 1973.

Lettin, Alan: Surgical treatment of low back pain. *Nurs. Times* 70: 1732–1735, 1974.

Lewis, H.L.: Who will regulate devices? Nurses and hospitals. *Mod. Hosp.* 121:74–76, November 1973.

Lloyd, H.M.: Fat embolism following multiple injuries. *Nurs. Times* 69:1490–1492, 1973.

Mallory, Thomas H.: *Total Care in Hip Replacement.* Warsaw, Indiana, Zimmer USA.

Marshall, John L.: Prosthetic cruciate ligaments: where do we stand?, *Orthop. Nurs. Assoc. J.* 3:37–39, February 1976.

Martin, Nancy; King, Rosemarie; and Suchinski, Joyce: The nurse therapist in a rehabilitation setting. *Am. J. Nurs.* 70:1694–1697, 1970.

Matzo, Lorraine: Nursing care — scoliosis surgery. *Orthop. Nurs. Assoc. J.* 2:251–255, October 1975.

Millender, Lewis H., and Nalebuff, Edward A.: Arthrodesis of the rheumatoid wrist. *J. Bone Joint Surg.* 55 [Am]:1026–1034, 1973.

Miller, Joseph E. [ed.]: Symposium: Bone Infections. *Clin. Orthop.* 96, October 1973.

Mooney, Vert; Cairns, Douglas; and Robertson, James: The psychological evaluation and treatment of the chronic back pain patient — a new approach. *Orthop. Nurs. Assoc. J.* 2:163–165, July 1975.

Moskowitz, E.: *Rehabilitation in Extremity Fractures.* Springfield, Ill.: Thomas, 1968.

Neufield, Alonzo: A ten minute examination to pinpoint skeletal injuries. *Orthop. Nurs. Assoc. J.* 2:273–274, November 1975.

Nute, Lois F., et al.: Nursing care of patients undergoing a total hip arthroplasty. *Orthop. Nurs. Assoc. J.* 3:43–54, February 1976.

O'Dell, Ardis J.: Hot packs for morning joint stiffness. *Am. J. Nurs.* 75:986–987, 1975.

Orthopedic Nurses' Association: *Home Care Manual.* Atlanta, Georgia, 1974.

Orthopedic Nurses' Association: *A Manual of Nursing Care Plans.* Atlanta, Georgia, 1975.

Patrick, Maxine: Little things mean a lot in geriatric rehabilitation. *Nursing '73*, pp. 7–9, August 1973.

Pavel, Alan, et al.: Prophylactic antibiotics in clean orthopaedic surgery. *J. Bone Joint Surg.* 56 [Am]:777–782, 1974.

Pendleton, Thelma, and Grossman, Burton J.: Rehabilitating children with inflammatory joint disease. *Am. J. Nurs.* 74:2223–2226, 1974.

Petrello, Judith M.: Temperature maintenance of hot moist compresses. *Am. J. Nurs.* 73:1050–1051, 1973.

Pigg, Janice: 50 helpful hints for active arthritic patients. *Nursing '74*, pp. 39–42, July 1974.

Pocock, Donald G.: Teaching patients — why and how? *South. Med.* 9–13, 70 1974.

Powell, M.: Limb traction — some aspects of nursing management. *Nurs. Mirror* 137:26–32, July 1973.

Roaf, Robert, et al.: *Textbook of Orthopaedic Nursing.* Philadelphia: Davis, 1971.

Robb, Susanne: Bunion surgery. *Am. J. Nurs.* 74:2181–2184, 1974.

Rockwell, Susan M.: Total hip replacement moves ahead. *R.N.* 35: OR/ED 21–24, May 1972.

Schmeisser, G.: *A Clinical Manual of Orthopedic Traction Techniques.* Philadelphia: Saunders, 1963.

Schneider, F.R.: *Handbook for the Orthopaedic Assistant.* St. Louis: Mosby, 1972.

Scott, Thomas F.: Total knee replacement nursing care. *Orthop. Nurs. Assoc. J.* 1:16–17, August 1974.

Shands, A.R., et al.: *Handbook of Orthopaedic Surgery* (8th ed.). St. Louis: Mosby, 1971.

Shoemaker, Rebecca: Total knee replacement procedure and results. *Nurs. Clin. North Am.* 8:117–125, 1973.

Simpson, Howard A.S.: Fractured femur and patella complicated by cerebral fat embolism. *Nurs. Times* 68:431–434, 1972.

Smith, C.: Osteomyelitis. *Nurs. Times* 70:862–865, 1974.

Sparks, Colleen: Peripheral pulses. *Am. J. Nurs.* 75:1132–1133, 1975.

Spickler, Linda: Fat embolism. *Orthop. Nurs. Assoc. J.* 2:146–147, June 1975.

Stein, Alice M.; Mandell, Delaine; and Ferguson, Jacqueline: Multiple fractures. *Nursing '74,* pp. 26–32, November 1974.

Stinchfield, Frank [ed.]: Symposium: Statistics on Total Hip Replacement. *Clin. Orthop.* 95, September 1973.

Stroup, Thomas E.: Traction techniques and special devices. *Orthop. Nurs. Assoc. J.* 1:86–87, November 1974.

Synnestvedt, Norwin [photographer]: The dos and don'ts of traction care. *Nursing '74,* pp. 35–41, November 1974.

Thomas, Betty J.: Total knee: New surgical miracle. *R.N.* 36: 35–39, September 1973.

Tronzo, Raymond G. [ed.]: Symposium on fractures of the hip. *Orthop. Clin. North Am.* 5(3): 571–583, 1974.

Tuomey, Sister M. Redempta: Halo pelvic traction. *Nurs. Times* 66: 1225–1228, 1970.

Viray, Primo: Nursing care in patients with a cervical spine injury. *Orthop. Nurs. Assoc. J.* 2:115–118, May 1975.

Warner, Thomas F.S.C., et al.: The cast syndrome. *J. Bone Joint Surg.* 56[Am]: 1263–1266, 1974.

Wells, Robert E.: Lumbar laminectomy and/or fusion. *Orthop. Nurs. Assoc. J.* 1:33–36, September 1974.

Williams, A.F.: *Guidelines to Orthopedic Nursing.* Missouri: Catholic Hospital Association, 1971.

Wilmot, A.: Total knee joint replacement. *Nurs. Times* 69:626–628, 1973.

Wishart, James: Fat embolism. *Nurs. Times* 67:1140–1141, 1971.

Works, Roberta F.: Hints on lifting and pulling. *Am. J. Nurs.* 72:260–261, 1972.

Young, Sister Charlotte: Exercise: How to use it to decrease complications in immobilized patients. *Nursing '75,* pp. 81–82, March 1975.

INDEX

Physical assessment—*Continued*
  equipment for, 2
  general vs. orthopedic, 2
  initial, in trauma, 31
Pillow
  in cast support, 187, 190
  in peroneal nerve palsy, 218
  splint, 31
  in turning patient, 151
Plantar flexion, defined, 4
Plantaris tendon rupture, 84
Plaster splints
  contour, 32
  use as partial casts, 187–188,
    189
Poliomyelitis, 134, 135
Polymyositis, 14
Polyneuritis, 136
Postoperative care. *See also
    specific topic, e.g.*, Femur,
    postoperative care
  explanation to patient, 194–195,
    196
  general, 196–197
  long-term goals, 196
  neurovascular evaluation of
    extremities, 155, 157–158
  transfusion, 195–196
Postoperative complications
  awareness of, 207
  compartment syndrome, 202–
    203, 205, 215–216
  decubitus ulcers, 163, 211–213
  fat embolism, 210–211
  osteomyelitis, 213–215. *See
    also* Osteomyelitis
  paralytic ileus, 216–217
  peroneal nerve palsy, 218–219
  prevention of, 198
  pulmonary embolism, 208–
    210
  thrombophlebitis, 207–208
  ulnar nerve traumatic neuritis,
    219
  Volkmann's ischemic con-
    tracture, 58, 216
Preoperative care, 194–196
  explanations to patient, 194–196
  osteomyelitis prevention and,
    214
  steroids in, 1, 196
Pressure dressings. *See* Elastic
    bandages
Progressive resistance exercise
    (PRE), defined, 225
Pronation
  defined, 3

measurement from neutral posi-
    tion, 4
Prosthesis
  femoral head, 72, 74, 217–218
  fitting after amputation, 207
Pseudarthrosis, congenital tibial,
    110, 111
Pulled elbow, 60, 62
Pulmonary embolism, 208–210
  high-risk patients, 208–209
  laboratory findings, 14, 209
  prevention, 208–209
  treatment, 209–210

Radial deviation, defined, 4
Radial nerve damage, 137, 232
Radius
  congenital absence, 110
  dislocations
    head, at elbow, 62, 63
    radiocarpal joints, 65
  fractures, 62, 63–64
    in children, 64
    Colles' fracture, 23, 41, 63–64,
      88
    head, 60
    reduction and fixation, 62, 63
  separation of distal epiphyses,
    64, 65
Range of motion (ROM), 3–10,
    11, 12. *See also specific
    topic, e.g.*, Ankle, range of
    motion
  congenital hyperlaxity, 110
  defined, 225
  degrees in recording, 4
  exercises. *See* Exercise;
    Exercise sling
  goniometer in measurement, 4, 5
  in history, 1
  neutral (anatomic) position of
    joint and, 4
  physical assessment of, 3–11
  right vs. left, 4
  rotation, 4
  terms, defined, 3–4, 225
Recurvatum. *See* Hyperextension
Rehabilitation, 45–46, 225–235
  after amputation, 207
  cane use, 233, 234
  crutches, 227–233. *See also*
    Crutch(es)
  discharge planning, 235–236
  education of patient and family,
    225, 233–235, 236
  exercise in. *See* Exercise(s)
  goals of, 45–46, 149–150

Thomas splint, 31
  in balanced suspension, 169,
    170
  in fractures, 82
Three-point gait on crutches,
    227, 228
Thrombophlebitis, 207–208
Thumb
  range of motion, 8
  tenosynovitis, 116
  trigger thumb, 144
Tibia
  bursting injury to, 86
  congenital absence, 110
  congenital pseudarthrosis, 110,
    111
  congenital torsion, 110
  epiphyseal injury, 86
  fractures, 82, 83
    in children, 84
    lateral and medial tibial
      plateaus, 81
    upper end, 83–84
  in knee dislocations, 81
  postoperative care, 202–203
  x-rays of, 20
Toe(s)
  congenital hallux varus, 110
  fractures and dislocations, 90
  range of motion, 11
Tomograms, described, 27, 28
Torticollis, congenital, 110
Torus fracture
  defined, 33–34
  of radius and ulna, 64
Total replacement of joints,
    131, 217–218
Traction
  alignment and countertraction,
    160–161
  balanced suspension plus, 169
  bedmaking and, 161
  CircOlectric bed and, 170, 221
  considerations and precautions
    in, 161, 162, 163, 164
  equipment for, 170–171
  examination of setup, 159–160
  explanation to patient, 194
  manual, described, 159, 163
  in neck injuries, 49, 205
  neurovascular evaluation of
    extremities in, 155, 157–
    158
  nursing care for patient in,
    161, 163
  overhead trapeze use in, 161

patient motility in, 161
  in pelvic fractures, 49
  peroneal nerve palsy and, 218
  pins in skeletal
    care of, 170, 171
    as infection site, 214
  prevention of decubitus ulcers
    in, 163, 212
  purposes and principles of,
    159, 163–170
  releasing or removing equip-
    ment, 161, 163
  skeletal, described, 159, 160
  skin, described, 159
  wedge Stryker frame and, 170,
    220
Transfer activities, 227, 235
Transscaphoid perilunate
    fracture-dislocation, 65
Trapeze. See Overhead trapeze
Traumatic arthritis, 131–132
Trigger thumb, 144
Trimalleolar fractures, 85, 86,
    87, 88
Trunk. See Chest; Pelvis; Spine
Tumors. See Neoplasms
Turning patient. See Moving
    patient
Two-point gait on crutches, 228,
    230

Ulna
  fractures, 62, 63–64
    reduction and fixation of, 62,
      63
Ulnar deviation, defined, 4
Ulnar nerve
  damage, 137
  postoperative traumatic neu-
    ritis, 219
Unicameral bone cysts, 121
Upper extremity. See Arm(s)
Urinalysis, 15

Valgus, defined, 4
Varus, defined, 4
Vertebrae. See Disc(s), inter-
    vertebral; Spine
Vitamin D-resistant rickets, 100,
    103
Volar compartment syndrome, 58
Volkmann's ischemic contracture,
    58, 216

Walker(s)
  exertion in use, 147–148